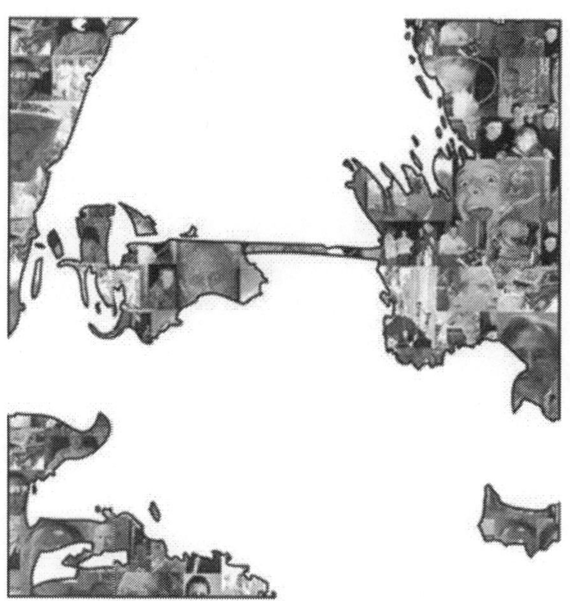

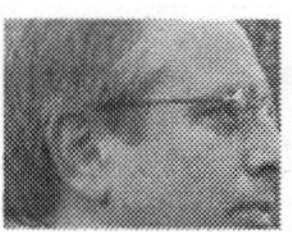

John C. Byler

with Laura Ricard, Ph.D

1 January 2012, Harvard, MA

Cataloging-in-Publication Data (for reference)

Byler, John C.

"You Look Great!" – Strategies for Living Inside a Brain Injury

Includes references and index.

1. Traumatic brain injury 2. Health and wellness. 3. Medical treatment strategies. 4. Relationships and community.

2012.

Abstract: *"You Look Great!"* presents The TBI Recovery Model, an interdisciplinary approach to recovering from a brain injury. The model's two checklists – Medical and Rehabilitation – help doctors and case managers answer the question, "Why do I feel so terrible all the time?" The book describes the role of each major medical and rehabilitation professional that should be considered as a referral to the TBI Recovery Team. With its personal narratives and strategy-session highlights with world-class specialists, *"You Look Great!"* narrows the gap between patients and the professionals who work with them; between patients and the caregivers and loved ones who live with them. The book is stocked with professional viewpoints, personal narratives and case studies, showcasing the clinical and very personal aspects of the brain-injury recovery process.

It is amazing!! This is going to sound weird, but this is the best way I can explain what I am feeling. I want to eat your book, devour it, have it part of me. I am slowly reading it. It's like a textbook for me. I am highlighting the same things I have felt and said. WOW!!!! I almost want to cry, because so far it is perfect. I wish I could read it faster. You have hit the nail on the proverbial head.

I am so happy you took the time to do this and to get input from other survivors. That there are people out there like me (to a degree) and that can understand makes me feel not so lonely and not so 'weird.' This book should be at every rehab hospital in the waiting rooms for families and friends of the survivors. Honestly, I adore this book!!!!

Kara Hoban, Pittsburgh PA

Should be required reading for anyone in neurology or emergency medicine.

I had a decent understanding before your book but learned a lot from you. I know there are a lot of "walking wounded" from our adventures in Iraq and Afghanistan and for the most part these men and women have to travel to West Palm, about 90 miles to the VA. I want to expand our facility to offer the help that is needed right here as well as educate people as to what help they do need. I suspect there is a lack of education among health care pros as to the type of therapies needed and available. I may need your help; scratch that . . . I will need your help. It's amazing how one's life can change so quickly. Amazing people take bad changes and turn them into something positive and good. God has a plan and He is never late. Keep inspiring. You are making a deep and lasting impact in so many lives.

Joseph Eriksen, Board of Directors, Sunshine Physical Therapy Clinic, Vero FL

Mission Statement of The "You Look Great" Project:

To enrich the day-to-day lives of brain-injury survivors with strategies, and increase the possibilities of their recovery

To learn more about The "You Look Great" Project, go to www.tbistrategies.com

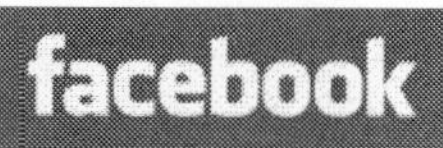

If you like what you see, make it official! "Like" the Project at Facebook.com/TheYouLookGreatProject

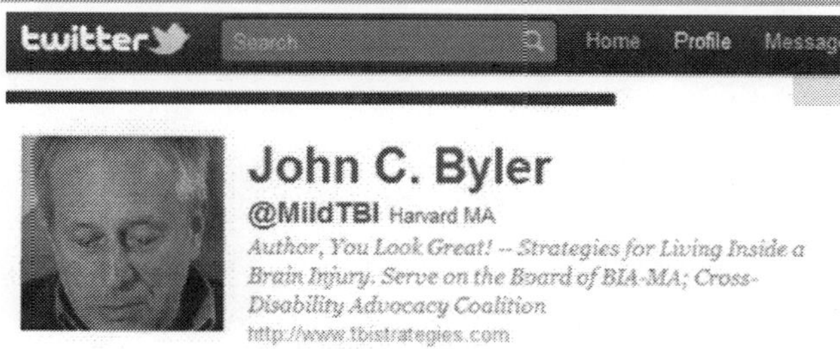

John is on Twitter @MildTBI for TBI-related tweets, and @ErasmusBlues for fun and penetrating insights into the human condition

To all those who live with a brain injury and are

determined to do more than simply survive it

To Lynne – you have been strong and brave,

understanding and wise. Thank you so much.

Table of Contents

Preface

> "I wish that I knew what I know now
> When I was younger.
> I wish that I knew what I know now
> When I was stronger."

From "Ooh la la," The Faces
(lyrics by Ronald David Wood, Ron Lane)

ABOUT THIS BOOK

Beginnings

In a way, this book began on YouTube. During the spring and summer of 2008, my filmmaker son Chris shot and edited a 55-minute video of a speech I have presented to graduate students and medical professionals in the Boston area. The video "You Look Great! – Inside a Traumatic Brain Injury" throws open a window into the not-well-understood world of neurotrauma rehabilitation.

My new friend Marilyn Spivack, founder of the Brain Injury Association of America and now neurotrauma coordinator for Spaulding Rehabilitation Hospital in Boston, wrote:

> This short film is a must-see for anyone whose life touches mild TBI: survivors, families, friends, and professionals. With great insight, courage, and humor, John gives us a rare view of what it's like to live with this injury. His story, images, and metaphors open up a world typically closed, invisible, ignored, or misunderstood.

This and many other enthusiastic responses *(Appendix A)* have been very encouraging of course, but they have also made me realize the urgency of writing this book. My thought was, if they like the video, they're going to love the book. Sure enough, as I began showing excerpts to fellow survivors, they all said pretty much the same thing: "I wish I'd had this book right after my injury."

Goal: Providing strategies to help TBI survivors

I am painfully aware of the need for clear, non-technical information about TBI and the recovery process. Most survivors and their caregivers are bewildered and desperate to know more about this injury and what lies ahead. If something like this book had existed in 2005 when I sustained my injury, I believe my recovery would have been more endurable and more complete. I would have felt less alone, clearer about what might be ahead for me, and used strategies other survivors had developed.

The lack of such a resource drove me to write this book. This book describes in detail what other survivors and I have learned about living with a brain injury. With its very personal narratives and rehabilitation strategies, I am confident that this book will help fellow survivors reduce the number of terrible days and in so doing help facilitate their recovery.

My street credentials

I have no formal education in neuroscience or medicine but I have a vast amount of excruciating field experience. This book avoids technical jargon and clearly explains most aspects of the injury and recovery in an accessible way.

I've kept extensive notes on the whole rehab and recovery process from the time of my injury in September 2005. I share what I've learned from my recovery team at Spaulding Rehabilitation Hospital in Boston, one of the top rehabilitation hospitals in the U.S. I have made plenty of mistakes that you can learn from and have had some breakthroughs that might help you.

You don't have to be in the NFL or WWF, a Golden Gloves champ, a soldier, or embedded journalist to suffer a brain injury. Brain injuries are democratic – anyone can get one. In fact, every 21 seconds, someone in the U.S. suffers a TBI. That's roughly 1.7 million people annually, with 52,000 of them resulting in death.[1] The fatalities are certainly tragic, and so are the lives of many of the survivors.

Many brain-injured people are walking around looking exactly as they did before their injury, but are undiagnosed and suffering beneath the surface. How could someone who "looks great!" – the most common compliment we get – have a brain injury? This book explains all that.

What this book provides

- Personal accounts of ongoing rehabilitation and recovery from mild and not-so-mild traumatic brain injuries

- What caregivers and other professionals should and shouldn't do when trying to help somebody recover from a brain injury

- Strategies for survivors: TBI patients do not often have "good days," only days that are less bad than others. To minimize the frequency of those truly awful days, we must use strategies we learn from neurotrauma and brain-injury specialists, as well as fellow survivors who are able and willing to share what they've learned along the way, about what helps and what can be disastrous

<u>Note</u>: Appendix B describes this book's intended audience.

Creating safe spaces for survivors

Survivors find it very hard to explain what a brain injury feels like. In part that is due to the uniqueness of brain injury from person to person. But it is also true that survivors talk in shorthand to each other, often cutting each other off with, "*You* know what I'm talking about." I don't know if you've ever been in a bar where combat veterans share an exclusive language that the rest of us can only guess at.

Because my goal is to provide an honest account of life inside a brain injury, I had to provide some detail into how it actually feels. Most TBI survivors feel strangely comforted to hear that others share their periods of misery. I wanted to reflect that reality, knowing the risk that it might sound like whining.

But we need to be clear with each other that complaining about one's injury survivor to survivor happens in a no-whine zone, a space that recognizes the difference between whining and communicating. We have to feel safe to talk about the discomforts and devastations of our injury with each other because:

- Knowing all that we have in common makes us feel less alone in all of this.

- It gives our loved ones and caregivers a bit of a reprieve from listening to us talk about the most fascinating, powerful thing that has ever happened to us.

THE BOOK'S ORGANIZATION

Recognizing the classic stages of grief – Shock, Anger, Rejection, Acceptance – is an important aspect of the grieving process. Knowing that these stages are normal for someone hard-hit by grief allows the afflicted to anticipate and then try to work through each highly interconnected stage.

TBI survivors and their caregivers work through a similar process. Because I believe that TBI survivors have three main phases in their recovery, I've organized this book into three sections:

- Awareness (of the injury)

- Adjustment (to the injury)

- Acceptance (of the injury)

Many of us become gradually **aware** of the injury after asking the profound and agonizing question, *"What is happening to me?"*

Through painful trial and error we then are forced to **adjust** our lives in countless ways, both small and large.

There then comes a period of time full of milestones marking our new lives of injury, and we come to **accept** that this has happened to us. Coming to this stage of acceptance can mean the difference between despair and hope, and sometimes the difference between a kind of death and a new way of living.

The purpose of this book is to facilitate adjustment and acceptance by raising awareness for survivors, their caregivers and medical professionals. A higher level of TBI awareness will reduce the floundering many survivors and their families experience in the early stages of TBI, and that many medical professionals experience as well when treating patients.

AWARENESS

"You are only coming through in waves.

Your lips move but I can't hear what you're saying . . .

I can't explain, you would not understand.

This is not how I am."

From Pink Floyd's "Comfortably Numb"
(lyrics by Roger Waters and David Jon Gilmore)

1 – Bagpiper on the Highway

WHAT YOU WOULD HAVE SEEN THAT NIGHT

If you'd been driving along the highway that night, you'd have thought they were shooting a movie. Southbound traffic suddenly crawled, and eventually on the grassy median, inside a barricade of three sets of flashing lights – fire-truck, ambulance and state trooper – you see an old blue Volvo rammed against an embankment, its trunk crushed into the back seat.

Not far from the wreckage you see a tall teenage boy playing the bagpipes. Three firemen surround him, grinning as they train their walkie-talkies on him, his blaring drones, and the melancholy wail of the pipes. The kid stood there as casually and coolly as if he were playing for dollar bills in Harvard Square, which he often did when he needed the money.

The man standing off to the side watching all of this, forehead in hand, trying to take it all in, was me, his Dad. Andrew didn't know it yet but he'd sustained three spinal fractures in his lower back. And I didn't know it yet but I'd suffered a traumatic brain injury.

THE BACK STORY

Once a week, either my wife Lynne or I drove our second son Andrew to his bagpipe band practice from our home in Harvard, Massachusetts to Wilmington, a 45-minute drive. On September 21, 2005 at about 9:15 p.m., Andrew and I were cruising home in the middle lane at about 65 mph on I-495 in my 1993 Volvo 240. We were listening to a Red Sox game – third-baseman

Bill Mueller was at bat – when, without warning, something slammed us from behind so hard we careened all over the highway.

It took long seconds for me to get control of the car as I shouted, "Oh my God! Oh my God!" In the panic of those seconds my windshield looked about a foot wide. If a car had been to our left as we went into the fishtail, that probably would have been the end of this story. But somehow we came to a full stop on the slope of the left-hand median strip between south- and northbound traffic. Andrew was the calm one. "Dad, are you okay?"

"Yeah, are you okay?"

"Yeah, I'm fine . . . Dad, are you sure you're all right?"

I guess he asked me a few times because he had never heard me shout like that. We got out of the car and saw the trunk accordioned into the backseat.[2] That's saying something because the 1993 Volvo 240 is built like a small tank.

I called 911 and then Lynne. My head hurt but I didn't have a mark on me. Andrew had a gash on his knee from ramming it into the dashboard, but aside from some jitters and aches we both seemed fine.

A UPS 18-wheeler pulled onto the median and the driver asked if we were alright. He must have seen the whole thing from a long way back. Another man ran over, crossing three lanes of traffic to get to us. He said he was a nurse and asked if we were all right. He pointed up the opposite side of the highway at the gold Mercedes that had hit us. A state trooper was already there talking to the driver.

An ambulance arrived. Two EMTs stepped out and asked me the usual what-year-is-this and who's-the-president questions. Then, "Do you want to go to the ER?" I double-checked with Andrew that he was okay and, because I felt overwhelming relief that we were both alive, I told them thanks, but no. We were going to be okay.

Months later, given how that night changed my life, I asked my Case Manager if we should have gone to the ER. She said that since I wasn't bleeding, hadn't blacked out, and could carry on a conversation, they would have given me two aspirins and sent me home.

Officer Miranda and the bagpipe fans

It's easy to remember the state trooper's name: Miranda, as in the you-have-the-right-to-remain-silent Miranda Rights. He asked me, "What happened?"

I pointed across the highway to the guy in the Mercedes and asked, "What did *he* say happened?"

"He said you'd come to a complete stop in the middle lane."

My jaw dropped, and Miranda said with total scorn, "I know. He's an idiot." He made notes on what really happened, and then went to his car to write his report.

It took me a year to talk about what happened next without choking up. As traffic roared past us, and firefighters and EMTs all milled around us, we were surrounded by the bright flashing lights of the fire-truck, ambulance and state trooper car. Men from the Chelmsford Fire Department asked if we wanted to retrieve anything from what remained of the car. I'd mentioned that I had a full tank of gas so they wanted to walk us over with a fire extinguisher. I said, "Yeah, Lynne's birthday present and Andrew's bagpipes."

It turned out one of the firemen was a huge fan of bagpipes – "I was just listening to bagpipes in my car!" – and he started asking Andrew questions about his piping band and that coming Saturday's Highland Games competition. In the midst of all that chaos, he then asked Andrew if he'd play something. He said sure, then he opened his case, put the pipes together, and played a gorgeous, powerful medley. The firemen trained their walkie-talkies on him so the guys back at the firehouse could hear him, too. He's played since he was 12 and by 16 he had gotten really good – I mean beyond his years good. If the pipes are played right – as he played them that night – they can be at once celebratory and funereal, joyful and melancholy, beatific and soulful.

After Andrew finished and we climbed into the cruiser, Trooper Miranda turned his siren on and, with his lights still flashing, edged his way into oncoming traffic. In the backseat, Andrew and I looked at each other, astonished, as he navigated us across the highway. He dropped us off at a rest area directly across from the accident, where Lynne was waiting for us. As Andrew and I got out of Miranda's patrol car and walked toward her, we saw the guy that hit us.

The perp walks

He looked like somebody out of Central Casting, if you were casting a movie about the Hell's Angels. He was limping. We made eye contact but he didn't say a word to us. He didn't say "sorry" or ask "how are you guys?" Nothing.

I only saw him that one time, but I've wondered since if he has been told what Andrew and I have been through. If he had beaten us with a baseball bat and we sustained the same injuries, they would have handcuffed him and he would probably be in prison for assault. For whatever reason – and the reason why he was not imprisoned was explained to me a few times and I still don't get it – he was free to go home. Something about having a valid driver's license and no evidence of being drunk.

Late that night

After we got home I was still shaken, but grateful that Andrew and I were still alive. I stared at the ceiling that night in bed, amazed that I lay there breathing next to Lynne, and that Andrew and his younger brother Will were sleeping peacefully in their beds down the hall. Our eldest son Chris had just started his first year of college; I was glad to imagine him at that moment reading a book or hanging out with some new friends.

I've been told that the Mercedes had to have been going over 100 miles an hour to flatten the back of a 1993 Volvo 240 cruising along at about 65 miles an hour. I shudder to think of what might have been, with all the heavy truck traffic across three lanes of I-495. I learned later that state troopers refer to this stretch of highway as Death Alley. When we sing about grace in church I think about us in that Volvo, delivered safely to the median strip by God and Swedish engineering.

As I said, Andrew fractured his back in three places, an injury that has not healed. He lives with constant pain. His brain is fine, although he too had a concussion and some lingering post-concussive symptoms. This led his pediatrician to impart this wisdom: "The reason you and your Dad are recuperating at a different pace has to do with brain plasticity. Your brain is veal and your Dad's is roast beef." (I have since learned that the reverse might also be true. Because a young person's brain is more malleable and still in the formative stages of development, an injury might have a more lasting and serious impact than an adult might experience.)

I often think about those bagpipes that night. Pipers traditionally perform at ceremonies that commemorate a beginning, like a wedding, or an end, like a funeral. Andrew's performance on the median strip next to our crumpled car looked and sounded like the happy conclusion of a close call. We couldn't guess about the grim battlefield ahead.

TBI AS FINGERPRINT

Now that you know the backdrop of my particular "incident," the rest of the book elaborates on what it's like to sustain and try to recover from a traumatic brain injury. In addition to testimony from other survivors I've interviewed, I describe in detail what many doctors and even neurologists don't know. I'm not being cocky here. You will read about some serious blind spots in the medical field about TBI, but the voices of survivors are being heard louder and clearer.

What survivors discover is that the human brain is so complex that its injuries are as specific and personal as a fingerprint, but far more intricate. So intricate – at the neuron level, in fact – that it is no wonder many brain injuries are so frequently misdiagnosed, or not diagnosed at all.

Traumatic brain injuries can also be debilitating, in a bizarrely ironic way. Take my new friend Gregg the firefighter, injured when the metal nozzle of a fire hose fell from the top of the fire-truck onto the top of his head. Gregg's internal gyroscope is so messed up – he can suffer such vertigo – that he can't climb a ladder. We survivors, veterans in this battle together, can chuckle about the irony, but nobody else probably should.

Although some of our symptoms overlap, my injury is different from Gregg's. For example, mine prevents me from easily organizing and sorting not only physical things but also ideas and information, which was a big part of what I did for a living for 25 years as an Instructional Designer. If I am talking without a script, I easily bog down because it's hard for me to sort through ideas and select words, which often ends in confusion and stammering.

Considering the respective injuries of a firefighter and a writer, it's easier, healthier I guess, to say that the injury can be ironic than to say it's cruel. Once you say it's cruel, finger-pointing and recriminations are not far behind, and recovery can begin to flag and even reverse itself when bogged down with attributing blame.

I am not being arrogant when I say that neurologists young and old, and even *summa cum laude* from Harvard Medical School, don't know a lot of what is in this book. If our brain injuries are like our fingerprints, then only we can describe every line and crack and whorl. And if the process of neurotrauma rehabilitation were common knowledge among neurologists, if it were at all predictable the way, say, recovering from an appendectomy or knee surgery usually has a predictable trajectory, my early treatment and that of other survivors would have been different, and we believe our recovery would have been faster and more complete.

So I don't get nervous when I speak with my prepared remarks in front of doctors, case workers, or graduate students in training. As someone recovering from a brain injury, I am often revealing information that they couldn't possibly learn elsewhere.

2 – Three Survivors
"Knocked into Another Dimension"

MIKE

"I realized that something was wrong, but I didn't know what."

Falling through the floor

At the time of his accident, Mike was a young, highly successful businessman. As he checked out some work a building contractor was doing for him, Mike fell through the flooring to the story below, landing on his back.

He spent three days in a hospital immobilized on a backboard. He had several bulging disks in his spine and had severely sprained his back. For more than a month he suffered extreme pain and did almost nothing except rest in bed. He vaguely remembers the events of the Christmas season swirling around him, but he mostly slept and watched television. "I wasn't doing anything. I was really just lying down." If he did get up to walk, he had to use a cane.

Because he did nothing during that first month of recuperation, Mike didn't have the opportunity to notice the damage to his brain. Other people saw his difficulties right away:

> They noticed that my speech had changed. I was stuttering. They told me that my speech was choppy and I wasn't calling people by their right names. My family also noticed. I realized that something was wrong, but I didn't know what.

The following day he sought help from his primary care physician, who then referred him to a neurologist.

Getting lost and sleepless nights

Before his appointment with the neurologist, new symptoms began to surface. He suffered a "tremendous amount" of double vision, seeing multiple images of single objects. To his alarm he began to get lost, the first time when he drove to his office – a trip on two main highways that he'd made many times:

> Not only did I forget the exit number; nothing looked familiar to me. That's terrifying. You can't believe it's happening. I don't remember exactly how I found my way to the office that day, but the problem continued. I would have situations where I left my office, which is normally a 25-minute commute, and 50 minutes would pass by and I would have no idea where the hell I was.

Mike's double vision would come and go, and if it happened while he was driving, he would pull over and cover one eye until his normal vision returned. Sometimes his surroundings would look completely alien, and he couldn't find his way home or to work. He bought a GPS for his car and became "100 percent reliant on it to find my way around."

The GPS got him back and forth to work, but his ongoing confusion caused him a lot of anxiety. He asked himself, *"Am I experiencing some type of dementia? Is the injury getting worse?"*

It is important to note that for many survivors, their lack of proper diagnosis intensifies their confusion and frustration. As you might expect, worsening symptoms can trigger a downward spiral of more confusion and fear.

Compounding his misery, Mike had real trouble sleeping. "It was like my circadian rhythm was off. My body didn't want to adhere to a normal sleep-wake schedule. If I let my body do what it wanted, it fell asleep at 3 or 4 A.M. I'd sleep for three hours from that point." His exhaustion aggravated all his other symptoms.

Diagnosis and getting help

The neurologist ordered a neuropsychological test and "that's when my doctors knew that something was seriously wrong." The neurologist told Mike that he'd sustained a very serious injury to his brain. He added that the injury was something that a lot of medical professionals "don't have experience with." Mike's primary care physician and the neurologist suggested that as a result of his fall Mike had probably suffered a concussion or was experiencing "post concussion syndrome."

The neurologist referred him to a highly regarded rehabilitation hospital, where a doctor finally diagnosed Mike with TBI:

> It wasn't until I saw the doctor at the rehab hospital that I really knew what was wrong. He explained what had happened and what TBI was . . . I had heard concussion and post-concussion syndrome and I'd think okay, I'm gonna be fine; it's just gonna be a little bit of time.

Mike was confident that this doctor "knew his stuff" because he worked at an institution staffed by "the best of the best." He thought that the doctor would "do what he needs to do and I'll be okay." Believing that he was in very good hands, he assumed that he would recover.

With this initial diagnosis, Mike could then begin work on clarifying and informing this sense of Awareness. As we will see, he is still working on Adjustment and, as with most survivors, the elusive Acceptance.

GREGG

"I couldn't walk. I felt the worst I'd ever felt in my whole life. It's hard to explain. It felt like the worst flu you could imagine."

An old hose with a brass coupling

In 2005, a week before my car accident, professional firefighter Gregg was performing a routine hose testing with his colleagues in the firehouse. Done for the day, the men began stowing equipment, including a large-diameter feeder hose that ran from the hydrant to the fire truck. Gregg steadied himself to throw the hose on top of the truck where it would dry out once they were back at the fire station:

> It was an old hose with a brass coupling, and it was extra heavy. I tossed it up to the truck top and it bounced back and smashed me on top of my head. It hit me really hard and I was dazed and I was, "Oh my God!" I was rubbing my head and didn't realize that blood was pouring out.

The men had a hard time staunching the bleeding so they called for an ambulance. In the emergency room Gregg was "conscious and alert and oriented." Doctors sutured his head "in one spot, on top of my head left of the center," and discharged him. He didn't finish his shift, but he was able to drive himself home. It was his wedding anniversary, but he and his wife Diana had postponed their celebration because she was working. Gregg spent the evening quietly.

The injury's gradual onset

The next morning when he woke up, Gregg felt "horrible and disoriented and foggy." He also felt like he had the flu. As had been the case with Mike and me, the possibility of even a mild concussion did not enter his mind.

> I felt like I was invincible, so I went over to work on the house that Diana and I are living in now. We were doing some restoration work on it and I went over to paint, but I got really nauseous. I began to vomit and had very strong flu-like symptoms. I was also very dizzy.

Gregg can't remember if it was that day or the next, but Diana, a nurse, insisted that he call their primary care physician. Diana says, "I was then thinking maybe concussion, but I was also thinking maybe flu, only it wasn't flu season." Gregg's physician told him that he probably had a concussion, and said, "Go home and it should resolve itself in a few days." These words have since reverberated in Gregg's mind many times.

Gregg began to experience what he thought were bizarre symptoms. Colors seemed "brighter than normal" and when Diana was driving he found himself almost panicky that she would crash due to his distorted depth perception. Even good old American paper money looked unfamiliar, "like foreign currency," and he lost much of his sense of smell and taste. He returned to his primary care physician to describe his symptoms and the physician referred Gregg to a neurologist.

Incomplete and insensitive medical treatment

The neurologist ordered a CT scan and an MRI. When Gregg returned to learn the results of his tests, the neurologist said coldly, "You got a concussion. Your CT scan and MRI were normal."

"I didn't like him," Gregg says:

> He was so matter-of-fact and unhelpful. He didn't tell us what to do, and failed to explain how long my symptoms would persist. Diana was upset. She said to him, 'My husband is not the same person he was; maybe you should get a second opinion.' But he shrugged his shoulders. There was no follow-up, no, 'Don't do this or do that.' Nothing.

Gregg's sequelae worsened. (<u>Note</u>: "Sequelae" differ from "symptoms." Symptoms are the evidence you see during the first 48 hours after an injury. After that, the evidence of a brain injury is referred to as sequelae.)

A few weeks after his visit to the neurologist, Gregg returned to his primary care physician. "That guy was terrible," he told his physician bluntly. The physician referred him to a different neurologist, "a very nice woman" who gave him medication to help him sleep. Like Mike, Gregg was also experiencing terrible insomnia. The second neurologist told him that she thought it was a concussion, but was unable to tell him how long his sequelae might last.

Although he had already been living with his injury for a month, his condition grew even worse:

> I couldn't walk. I felt the worst I'd ever felt in my whole life. It's hard to explain. It felt like the worst flu you could imagine. With assistance

I walked out to the ambulance. I went to my wife's hospital where I got red carpet treatment. They gave me medication and said it was mostly migraine, but I'd never experienced any migraines. They gave me fluid.

So I went home and down into our cellar where I stayed on the couch. It was dark and quiet. I'd been down there three weeks when for about 24 hours there was a strobe-like effect in my eyes, and I'd drift off and, geez, is there a police car outside? I'd wake up wondering, is the strobe-like vision part of a migraine? It seemed too unusual to last that long.

I was disturbed. My symptoms continued, although now even my touch sense was affected. Things felt cold to my fingers.

Seeing specialists

Gregg was referred to another doctor, a sports-concussion specialist. Gregg described his sequelae, but the specialist didn't prescribe medication. In fact, he failed to prescribe any therapy at all. "He told me nothing about what to do and what not to do."

Gregg went to see the specialist a second time, and a month or so later returned to see him again. During this third visit Gregg complained of "oddball" symptoms. "I kept tripping over things and felt like I wasn't seeing things down below, as if my vision were cut off when I was walking on a sidewalk and going downstairs in my house."

As many survivors have told me, Gregg recalls that the specialist was "short" with him. "He threw up his hands and said, 'Well, I don't know why you're not getting better.'" He referred Gregg to a neurotrauma rehabilitation specialist and suggested that he also see an ophthalmologist for his vision problems. At this point, a full year into his injury, Gregg and Diana felt like they were "floundering."

As with Mike, they were certainly in the Awareness stage, knowing that something was wrong with Gregg's brain and body. But nobody could tell them what Gregg's injury was, how to treat it, or what to do next.

In the meantime, Diana researched brain injuries on the Internet and asked her colleagues at the hospital a lot of questions. Gregg recalls that some of their answers upset her:

> She was talking to another nurse and the nurse out of the blue said, "He won't get better." Diana just cried. She said to me, "How could she say that? It's not supportive." But the nurse was actually a nice person and had known people who hadn't recovered. That's why she said that. It was really hard for Diana to hear because at that point we always thought I'd fully recover.

It took Gregg another two years – three years after the accident – to realize that he was "never gonna be normal the way I was before the injury." Today, when he tries to explain what the injury feels like, he says, "It's like being knocked into another dimension."

TOM

"The ER doctor said nothing was wrong with me and told me to take it easy."

Tom worked as an outreach sales specialist for a large international bank headquartered in New England, and he loved his job. The bank has branch offices in a large chain of grocery stores, and Tom covered his sales territory in Western and Central Massachusetts, greeting store customers in the aisles and inviting them to do business with the bank. The job required a lot of self-confidence and an ability to work in a fairly chaotic environment.

Tom excelled at this work, and the bank soon named him "Salesman of the Quarter." Tom felt real pride in this recognition.

> It was a great job. For the first time I was making great money and really felt good about my life. It was rewarding, too. I got to meet a lot of people and build relationships with them.

The accident

The day after the award, he was driving to Boston for a mandatory staff meeting when another car hit him head-on. The collision smashed his neck's fourth vertebra. It took him a long time to figure out that the accident had also injured his brain.

Tom didn't lose consciousness, but he felt panicky – he had never been in a wreck and smoke filled the inside of his car. He dragged himself out through his window:

> The person who was driving behind me came to me to make sure I was okay. He wanted me to lie down, but I had my long cashmere coat on and it was important to me and I didn't want to ruin it. I made phone

> calls – I think I was probably delirious – to Arthur (my partner), my boss and my parents. I'm saying goodbye to them; I thought I was dying. I felt numb all over – I didn't know that the fourth vertebra in my neck had been smashed – and my knee hurt. I was in a daze.

The botched response of medical professionals

The ambulance arrived and the paramedic evaluated Tom's condition by asking him such questions as, "How many fingers am I holding up? Do you know your name?" The paramedic insisted that Tom go to the hospital, but Tom refused to budge until Arthur arrived. "The minute Arthur got out of his car he waved and I said to the medic, 'Okay, you can take me.'"

Even without previous exposure to the world of brain injury, Tom assumed that doctors at the hospital would order an MRI or a CT scan, but all they did was take an X-ray. "The ER doctor said nothing was wrong with me and told me to take it easy."

The aftershocks

At first, Tom and Arthur focused on Tom's physical problems. The crushed disc in Tom's neck was painful; it didn't occur to either of them that his brain might have been injured. Then, about a month after the accident Tom began to show signs of emotional distress. He cried easily for no apparent reason and had acute anxiety:

> I needed to isolate myself so I retreated to a back bedroom in our house where I just sat in a chair and stared out the window. I didn't want to get into the car to drive to the doctor because I felt petrified. It was weird: Sound bothered me, and I had a feeling that's hard to explain. It was like I wasn't comfortable in my own skin.

> I had panic attacks at night and night sweats. The panic attacks were so bad I had to get up and walk around and sometimes I had to run up and down the stairs to try to release some of my stress. At times I couldn't breathe.

Like Mike and Gregg, Tom couldn't sleep. He'd go to bed, sleep a few hours, and then wake up and wander the house for the remainder of the night. (To this day the men's ability to sleep is seriously compromised.)

Over the next few weeks he continued to experience severe anxiety attacks, and his night sweats got so bad that he had to change the sheets two or three times a night. He also experienced disconcerting surges of energy:

> That first weekend I went into the kitchen and rearranged everything – all the dishes and pots and pans and glasses. My partner couldn't find a thing. I felt so much energy that I cleaned the fish tank out too, but I forgot to acclimate the tank water. So now I'm tired and exhausted, I didn't sleep, I just tossed and turned, and when I went down to feed the dogs I noticed all the fish were dead.

Tom snapped when he saw all the dead fish. He dropped to the floor and screamed, "What's going on?" Arthur had been in the mental-health field for years and understood immediately that Tom was behaving clinically manic – highly excitable with bursts of energy and rage. Thoroughly frightened, he told Tom, "We need to see someone and we need to see someone *now*." Arthur made an appointment with Tom's primary care physician.

Tom told his primary care doctor about the accident, who then asked him if he had lost consciousness. "When I told him no, he fluffed it off. He pooh-poohed it." Tom added that he felt depressed and anxious, and "without even digging deeper," the doctor put him on Prozac. Tom began to take the Prozac, but his anxiety grew so much worse that the doctor changed his medication to Zoloft.

Zoloft made Tom's anxiety even worse. "It didn't calm me down or relax me or stabilize my mood. I couldn't focus. I was a mess."

The primary care doctor did not even suggest that Tom have an MRI, which would have revealed Tom's serious neck injury, and it never occurred to Tom to request a referral to a neurologist or any other specialist. Arthur recalls, "We were completely in the dark."

Five weeks later

Five weeks after the accident, Tom had used up his vacation and sick time for the year. Fearing that he would lose his job, he forced himself to return to work. It took him forever to get there because he experienced suffocating panic attacks in the car. The attacks were so intense that he had to pull off the road repeatedly. He cried all the way.

At work he found it impossible to talk to anyone and "shut down":

> The job had taken me out of my shell. I'd finally started living. Before the accident I found myself feeling good about standing in front of people and talking and giving presentations. I was passionate about what I did. Now I couldn't focus, think, or remember, and it scared me. And my colleagues treated me as damaged goods. They avoided me, big time.

Tom's sales numbers plummeted. "I couldn't sell. For this job you have to stand out there and talk to people and be assertive and I couldn't do it." The bank sent him to an eight-hour training class held in a windowless office.

Feeling suffocated, Tom could not control his anxiety. Observing his behavior, a colleague urged him to contact the employee assistance program (EAP).

Tom told the EAP agent everything. "I started from Day 1 with the accident, my breakdowns, the night sweats, the panic attacks and my anxiety about driving. I was also feeling claustrophobic all the time and feeling afraid, so I told her that too. The people with the EAP program thought there was something wrong with me upstairs. I knew it had something to do with the accident."

3 – Sudden Impact:
Not Just the Name of a B Movie

THE DEVASTATION OF AN INVISIBLE INJURY

What happened to Mike, Gregg, Tom and me occurs every day here in the U.S., to our troops who served and are serving overseas, and to countless others around the world. Other venues that can cause a TBI include the obvious – boxing rings, UFC cages and football fields at the professional and amateur levels – and the less obvious: a slippery sidewalk or standing up under an open file drawer. (*Note: Appendix C describes the prevalence and toll of TBI.*)

We survivors are all learning that too many members of the medical community are in the dark about TBI. This is especially true for so-called mild TBI; an MRI is not standard procedure if the survivor did not lose consciousness or does not display more obvious signs of brain damage. Researchers are just beginning to understand what TBI is, how to diagnose it, and how to minimize TBI damage when a blow leaves no immediate evidence. Understanding the injury is further complicated by its personal touches; survivors share many of the same sequalae, but not all and not to the same degree.

How is the brain traumatized?

The brain has the consistency somewhere between Jell-O and Silly Putty, and the inside of the skull that houses it is not lined with protective padding. The human skull is of course bone – and much of it is not even smooth bone, but ridged. Because the area behind the eyeballs, the orbitofrontal area, and the anterior temporal area are especially rough and bony, these areas are most susceptible to contusion in a TBI. So when the brain is violently shaken inside the skull it often crashes against a hard and hostile surface. Brain neurons can twist, stretch and even tear.

A survivor of brain trauma might be permanently disabled even though he or she looks great. Because neurons are so tiny – anywhere from four microns (.004 mm) to 100 microns (.1 mm) in diameter – their twisting and stretching, shearing and tearing do not show up on a CT scan, an MRI, or an EEG. Survivors with clean tests are usually said to suffer from only "mild" TBI.

"You can't fix what you don't see or understand"

Joseph, a friend of mine from high school, spent 30 years in Emergency Medical Services and still works on an ambulance. He writes:

> I have dealt with hundreds of head injuries and the most insidious are the TBIs. It is easy to splint a bone or medicate an ischemic heart. You can spot respiratory distress across a room and sometimes easily fix it. You can't fix what you don't see or understand. Also, in EMS you rarely follow a patient beyond delivery to the ER. But a good medic should always hold a high suspicion of TBI in any trauma involving the head.

Without a proper diagnosis – which eventually came – Mike, Tom and Gregg could not to move on to Adjustment. As these stories show, the inadequacy of diagnosis and treatment is part of the reason why TBI is devastating. As Gregg put it, TBI knocks its victims into another dimension.

4 – The First Week and Month of Injury

Woe to me because of my injury! My wound is incurable! Yet I said to myself, "This is my sickness, and I must endure it." My tent is destroyed; all its ropes are snapped." Jeremiah 10:19-20

THE FIRST WEEK

The next two chapters outline my first week, month and year of decline and only partial recovery. I include them so that other survivors can compare their stories and progress. These chapters illustrate that unlike, say, a knee or shoulder injury, the symptoms of a traumatic brain injury might unfold gradually but with frightening intensity. They certainly did in my case, and they did for Mike, Gregg and Tom.

It can take a week for the brain to register the awful impact of a collision – whether a car or a fist – and then communicate the damage to the rest of the body. In fact, the first seven days of a traumatic brain injury often follow their own complex timeline.

Day 1: Thursday, September 22, 2005

The morning after our accident – Thursday – I felt pretty rattled but collected myself for long enough to send an e-mail to some family, friends and colleagues about what had happened. It read like the story of a narrow escape.

I tried to make some progress on some work, but after an hour I had to stop. I was still shaken up and couldn't concentrate. I also felt very strange and leaden, like I had the flu, complete with aches and pains in my body.

My neck hurt and Lynne urged me to have it x-rayed, which I then did. The doctor on call at my GP's office said that, while she was not a radiologist, the x-rays looked okay to her. I felt like asking, "So, does your opinion count or not?" She prescribed a muscle relaxant. She said nothing about the possibility of a concussion or contracoup, a form of trauma as in the case of whiplash where the brain crashes into the front and back of the skull. She said nothing about how I should take care of myself, and nothing about what I should expect or do next.

I took the muscle relaxant in the evening and slept until very late Friday morning, rare for me because I usually didn't sleep in, even on weekends.

Day 2: Friday, September 23, 2005

On Friday, I attempted to work at my home office with the hopes of finishing up a project. Although I normally would have spent a half day revising it, I worked for about an hour but couldn't keep at it; I felt burned-out and depleted. I sent it off, feeling pretty confident that it was at least presentable.

When I sent the e-mail, I thought, "Now I have the weekend to recover."

My symptoms worsened and new ones reared their ugly heads. It is hard for many survivors to explain how they feel, other than to say "terrible." Though sharing some symptoms with the flu, I wasn't sweating, shivering, vomiting, or feverish. I felt as though I had been badly beaten up, although with only dull, generalized pain. I also had a powerful feeling of grief and cried easily for no reason. "Terrible" is a pretty good word to describe the overall feeling.

Any kind of stimulus – any light or sound – irritated me to the extreme, as though I had a complete-body hangover. Fortunately, I did not suffer migraines the way many survivors do. I retreated to the floor of our large bedroom closet, where I lay in the dark on a cushion and ended up sleeping all afternoon.

Day 3: Saturday, September 24, 2005

Saturday things fell apart. When I eventually woke up, I felt like I was moving in slow-motion.

I took my son Will to his baseball game and watched a few innings, but all I could think about was how awful I felt. Like many TBI survivors, I was completely in the dark about what was happening to me. To get away from the other parents, I walked over to the chain link fence and called our friend Holly, a doctor. I told her about the accident and how I was feeling, and after struggling with my words I leaned onto the fence and burst into tears.

She knew me well enough to know that I was acting oddly out of character. With her soothing and confident voice, she offered encouraging words about how, on the night of the accident, I had steered the ship into a safe harbor and that the whole experience must have been very traumatic for me. She assured me that I had acted heroically, and reminded me that both Andrew and I were now safe because I managed to get the car off the highway and onto the median.

Then she said my main symptoms sounded like post-traumatic stress, but that my stammering and inability to sustain a narrative concerned her. That didn't sound like post-traumatic stress to her. She said that I was showing "lability," an emotional fragility that led me to cry easily. She urged me to go to our local hospital Monday morning and get a CT scan.

I should note that I was fortunate to have had this advice. Some survivors do not have their brains examined for a very long time – even months or years – after their initial incident.

Day 4: Sunday, September 25, 2005

Before church on Sunday, the pastor announced my narrow escape to the congregation. Someone I didn't know leaned over to me and said that healing would take time and a lot of rest. For some reason that was a crazy tipping point because I stood up and ran outside and melted down in the parking lot. Lynne met me there and we stood there crying in each other's arms.

I don't know if you can tell from my workmanlike, dispassionate prose, but I'm not an emotional person. So what was happening to me? Lynne encouraged me to come back inside, so I did. After church a few people talked to me, wishing me well and telling me what they knew about concussions. They didn't know I was finding all of these interactions absolutely bewildering and surreal.

We went home and I spent the afternoon in bed sleeping. I also felt a suffocating dread about having to function like a normal human being the next morning, a Monday. It wasn't so much a question of performance; it was a matter of even hoping to carry on a normal conversation. I felt as if I had been jammed through a meat grinder.

Day 5: Monday, September 26, 2005

On Monday, things got worse. Recounting the accident on the phone to a close colleague, I got so distraught that I ended up holding my head in my hands and said, "I'm a f---ing wreck," a word not normally in my vocabulary. I told him that maybe if I just took the week off I'd be okay.

Then I remembered the phone meeting in an hour and a half that would kick off a new project. Usually, a call like that would have been kind of exciting for me, but I had no confidence in my ability to engage in a coherent conversation. I hated to do it, but I cancelled the meeting.

CT scan in the ER

That afternoon, due both to what Holly had said and to my progressively worsening ability to talk, Lynne called my primary care physician and told him everything. He said I should go immediately to the ER and get a CT scan.

I drove myself there because I didn't want Lynne to have to spend hours waiting for me. She had work to do – actual, billable hours. At some point, as the hospital's bureaucracy moved me through its system like an amiable kidney stone, they put me in a wheelchair. I sat in the hallway for a while, waiting for my turn in the CT scan room, sort of detached from the whole thing. I exchanged glances with doctors and nurses with a pleasant smile on my face as they hurried past, but I started to feel chagrined because I knew I didn't really need the wheelchair. That line from Pink Floyd's "Comfortably Numb" kept going through my head: "This is not how I am."

The CT scan was easy and quick. They moved me into another room to wait for the ER's Attending Physician to give me the results right then and there. I sat for quite a while on the butcher-paper wrapped padded table just looking around, and thinking about what on earth could be next. It also felt strange not to be working on a Monday afternoon.

Eventually the doctor breezed in and said, "Good news on your CT scan; there's no bleeding." Then he put me through an informal neuropsych test, which began with just trying to stand on one foot at a time. I struggled with that, which surprised me because I usually have pretty good balance. Then he said, "I'd like you to count backwards from 100 by sevens."

I had to ask him a few times to repeat the instructions, and when I felt I understood them I tried to do the math. "100 . . . 93 . . . uhh . . ." I was taking so long between each increment and struggled so mightily that his expression became serious and said I should make an appointment to see the hospital's neurosurgeon.

I thought, "A neurosurgeon? Don't they, like, cut people's heads open?" I wasn't in any kind of position or frame of mind to ask him why I should see a neurosurgeon, so I drove home and told Lynne everything. She called the neurosurgeon's office and made the appointment for Wednesday, one week after the accident.

Day 6: Tuesday, September 27, 2005

On Tuesday I slept a lot, and did as little as possible.

Day 7: Wednesday, September 28, 2005

A week after the accident, Lynne drove us to the hospital to meet with the neurosurgeon. While Lynne parked the car, I found the elevator and walked to his office, wishing she was with me, wondering how long she'd be. A woman at the desk behind the glass handed me some forms to complete and I just looked at her, totally confused. I asked her to explain what she meant and I couldn't follow her instructions, not to mention make sense of the forms in my hand.

Just then Lynne walked in and the woman told her, "He's had a concussion," which was news to me. I'd never had a concussion before and I didn't know anything about them. I knew I hadn't blacked out and, besides, the accident was a whole week ago. In movies if a guy gets karate-chopped on the back of the neck or slugged on the head with a pistol butt, he blacks out. And when he "comes to," he rubs his neck or shakes his head and tries to find the guy who did it.

Lynne filled out the paperwork for me. As we waited, I stared at all the framed photographs on the wall. Professional wrestlers, boxers and football players scrawled their gratitude to the man I was about to meet. I felt so out of place.

The neurosurgeon was wearing his blue surgeon's outfit for each of the five or six times I saw him. My meetings with this brain surgeon had to have been the most bloodless ones he would have all day. He wanted to hear everything. I started from the beginning, and in my new stop-and-start way of talking, mired in deep emotion, I told him about the accident; as I did so, he observed the symptoms.

He threw the neck x-ray up onto the vertical light box with an impressive slap, a practiced move, and pointed right away to my neck, noting the evidence of whiplash. As he conducted his own neuropsych test for me, I tried to stand on one foot and actually choked up and got teary as I tried again to count down from 100 by sevens. Seeing all of this, he said:

> I want you to go home and spend the next three weeks doing nothing: no mental or physical exertion of any kind. If it were up to me, you would lie in bed and stare at the ceiling.

More tears came when he said that, but why? They were probably due to a number of things but mostly I think they came from a place of relief. Because I looked fine on the outside and my brain wasn't bleeding, I had worried that he was going to dismiss me and tell me to just deal with it. How many football coaches or boxing managers tell their guys to get back in there? Instead, he was acknowledging that something serious was happening to me. And doing nothing was exactly what I felt I needed to do, or even all that I could do.

THE FIRST MONTH

Even doing nothing is doing a lot

What should you do in the first month after a brain injury?

As . . . little . . . as . . . possible. Keep the visual and auditory stimulation to a minimum! As one person put it, "Don't pick at the scab."

Most of the time nothing is all you feel like you can do anyway. But then you'll have a day when you don't feel so bad and you start thinking:

"Is it over? Am I better? Can I just do . . . this?"

And if you're still injured, you'll find out the answers:

Sorry, but no it's not over, no you're not better, and don't even think about exerting yourself because you'll burn out really quickly and feel like you're back at square one.

That's why doctors should not be releasing the brain injured back into the wild. To recover from a brain injury – or, more accurately, because we might not actually recover, to *facilitate healing* from a brain injury – you've got to rest your brain. That's the way it is for heart-attack patients; they've got to rest their hearts. A heart-attack patient wouldn't dream of trying to run around the block, work on his taxes, or bet on horses. A woman with a broken kneecap cancels her tennis game, and a guy with a dislocated shoulder won't even play touch football with his kids.

But here's our dilemma: part of recovering from a brain injury involves experimenting to see what you're still capable of doing. So you find out you can't read for more than, say, 15 minutes or only two minutes because you start feeling terrible. That's the test. It involves lots of trial and lots of error. The key is to learn from mistakes. Survivors who are stubborn and who are used to being high-performing have an especially hard time with the discipline of stopping an activity before feeling bad.

That first month, aside from feeling terrible most of the time, my brain felt like it had been tightened, and that it was "full" . . . like after a Thanksgiving dinner. I didn't want to put anything else in it. I couldn't read or even listen to music.

It occurred to me then that every time we open our eyes or even hear something we are processing information – even when we're doing something like sitting in the backyard looking at trees. And so, especially early on in our recovery, those of us with a brain injury need to have down time from our down time.

In the movie "The Matrix," Neo could see the world as it really is: lines upon vertical lines of green code raining down. Our brains receive the world as information. With my eyes open and my eardrums tender, I found that the world of information crashed into my brain, and my brain worked hard to process it. Sometimes it shut down completely, the way a lawnmower shuts down when you run over a patch of really long grass.

So for the next ten days I basically sat out in the back yard on a bench swing all bundled up. Through dark sunglasses I watched the trees slowly change color. This was, after all, autumn in New England.

I often watched distant airplanes leaving white streams that would fade into the blue sky. I thought, "That's what my memory is like." And then one day as I lay perfectly still, under piles of blankets, the biggest hawk I've ever seen flew over and landed on top of the swing. He stayed there for about 20 seconds and I felt blessed.

Looking great while doing puzzles

Family, friends and colleagues sent me cards and some called the house asking about me. Of course, we had moments of misunderstanding. Because I sat outside doing nothing, I developed a tan and people said, "Hey, you look great!" That beats the alternative, for sure. Without seeming defensive, I tried to explain that even though I looked the same, my brain was sort of in traction.

Every once in a while someone would say something awkward, like, "What I wouldn't give for some time off" or "Our son had five concussions." I knew they meant well but I never knew how to respond, what with fluency being one of my biggest challenges.

As the days wore on my symptoms persisted. The tinnitus – ringing in ears – and hyperacusis – sensitivity to noise – were mostly just annoying because my bigger concerns included short-term memory, language and a deadening fatigue. I couldn't hold onto a simple arithmetical calculation or the letters in someone's name as he repeated them to me over the phone so I could write it down.

I couldn't formulate responses to such simple questions as, "How are you feeling?" One Saturday morning my brother called simply to ask how I was doing. I stammered so badly I became incoherent, and the cognitive effort devastated me through the next day.

For some reason I enjoyed putting together colorful 300-piece puzzles, maybe because I wasn't reading yet. Using my hands felt good, but a lot of it had to do with taking the chaos of the puzzle pieces and putting them all together. I think it served as a hopeful metaphor for putting my brain back together.

Figure 1:

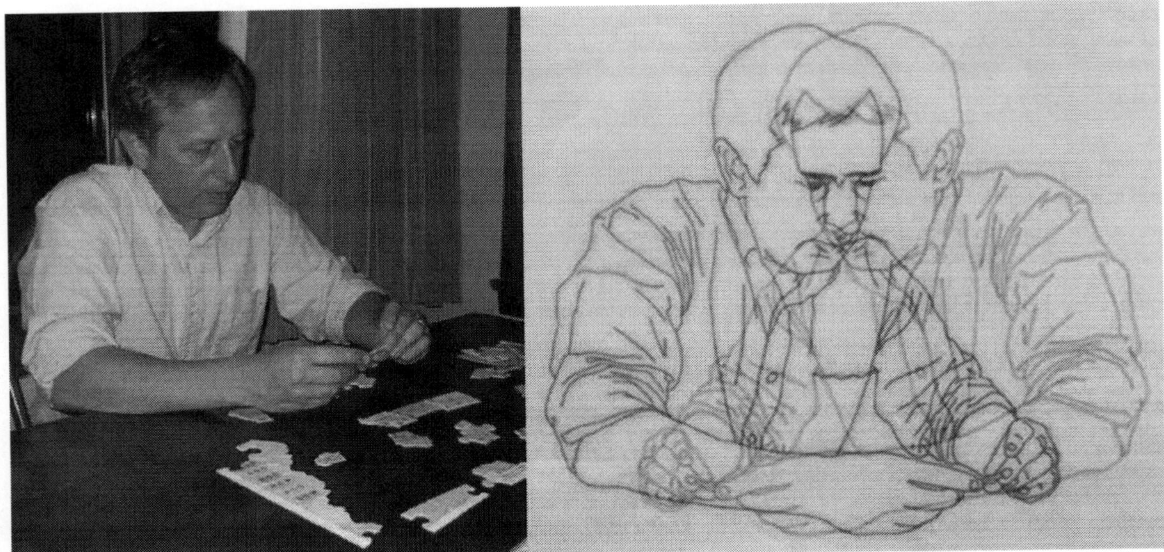

<u>*Artist*</u>*: Joshua Caleb Weibley*

And meanwhile, I was missing big parts of my life, like my youngest son Will's two out-of-the-park homeruns.

Missing work

Besides the obvious physical toll the injury exacted on me, I also felt badly about missing so much work. It wasn't guilt I was feeling because the injury was clearly out of my control, but somehow I still felt I was letting my colleagues down by not healing faster. I hammered out an e-mail explaining my absence and added:

> I've been told to only worry about getting better . . . so I'll just take one thing at a time. This includes putting together some pretty great puzzles, listening to Frank McCourt read *Angela's Ashes*, and I'm allowed to take walks now so I've been seeing the autumn trees with completely new eyes. And that's not a bad thing.

I also fretted that my employer wouldn't want me back if I was damaged goods. They hire only the best and the brightest, and now I was neither.

Re-scheduling and then finally getting the MRI

Two weeks into the three weeks of non-activity the neurosurgeon had prescribed, Lynne called his office to say that not only was I not getting better, but I seemed to be getting worse. He had her schedule my MRI for that night.

On the way there, she asked if I was nervous, and never having had an MRI before, I said no. I changed into one of those embarrassing little johnnies and hopped up on the table. The nurse asked if I was ready, and, thinking it would be like the CT scan, I said sure. I lay down and she gave me a rubber thing to squeeze if I wanted to come out of the MRI tube. She placed my head flat and put a cage over my face. As I started moving into the MRI tube I looked around and felt like I was being slid into a casket. I panicked so I squeezed the rubber thing and shouted, "I can't do this!"

My panic was another by-product of the injury. I could no longer cope with all sorts of problems that came up, whether physical, mental, or emotional.

I walked sheepishly back into the waiting room and we left without completing the scan. Lynne rescheduled me for the next day, but this time I would take Valium. That evening, anticipating the intense claustrophobia ahead, I read a Psalm that seemed addressed to me. It made me smile because I thought it was so specific. Psalm 139 became my MRI Psalm. It begins:

> O Lord, you have searched me and you know me.
> You know when I sit and when I rise; you perceive my thoughts from afar.

> You discern my going out and my lying down; you are familiar with
> all my ways.
> Before a word is on my tongue you know it completely O Lord.
> You hem me in – behind and before; you have laid your hand upon
> me.
> Such knowledge is too wonderful for me, too lofty for me to attain.
> Where can I go from your spirit?

Certainly not inside an MRI tube. (<u>Note</u>: I have put together some tips for getting through an MRI in Appendix E.)

The MRI results revealed no apparent brain damage, but the neurosurgeon noted my lack of progress. He actually used the word "regress." He had us schedule a sleep-deprived EEG to examine my brain circuitry. I was to stay awake all night and show up first thing in the morning. "Another piece of the puzzle," he called it. He remained confident that I would fully recover, which Lynne and I mentally filed away, at peace with his confidence.

"Most people would have gotten better by now"

The EEG itself was a breeze. The hardest part was the staffer interview beforehand when I stammered and had memory lapses. The neurosurgeon reported that the results of this test also showed no problems. I took this as good news, but I wasn't prepared for what happened next. He said, "Most people would have gotten better by now," which made it sound like my lack of progress – my regression – was my fault. I thought he sounded annoyed, and disappointed in me.

How could I explain to him that I would do anything to feel better? I told Lynne later in the parking lot that he was really at a disadvantage because he didn't know me before the injury. He didn't know about my facility with words, my ease around other people, my confidence speaking to groups of 250 people, or about my pride in my work and reputation among colleagues. How could he know how different this man sitting there in his office really was, suddenly inarticulate and emotional? He then explained that there was nothing surgically for him to do. He gave me two options:

- Do nothing, and let nature take its course (I thought later, "Yeah, we all know how reliable nature can be"), or

- See Beth Adams, a neurotrauma rehabilitation expert who specializes in evaluating cognitive skills and developing the coping and problem-solving skills that help brain-injured people try to lead as normal a life as possible.

I was kind of shocked. I thought but did not say, "But a rehab expert isn't a doctor! Are you saying there's nothing doctors can do for me now . . . that there's no doctor who can help me?"

As I left his office, opting to see Beth as soon as possible, I felt confused and defeated. This neurosurgeon was a noted neurotrauma specialist, but this would be my last visit with him. The "answer guy" had done all he could with me and handed me off, just as Gregg's doctor, and the doctors of many other survivors I have spoken with since, have done. As it turned out, seeing Beth was the absolute best next step for me, but more on all of that shortly.

5 – The First Year of Injury

THE SEQUELAE OF "MILD" TBI

As we've seen, survivors of mild TBI experience many of the same sequelae, but of varying intensities and durations. Sometimes the sequelae disappear entirely, and other times the intense, crippling sequelae persist for a lifetime.

I have urged survivors, "Go to the gym! Go running!" because vigorous, regular exercise happens to make me feel a little better. But some survivors, like Gregg, can't exercise because their injury includes vestibular issues that cost them their balance and often make them nauseous. As I said early on, Gregg is a former firefighter who can't climb a ladder because it makes him dizzy, and early on had days when he had to crawl around the house on all fours.

Doctors I've spoken with agree that the more physically active a survivor can be, the more blood will flow through the brain, which might facilitate its healing. The point here though is that although the sequelae of mild TBI survivors overlap, many are different and even the ones that are the same are really quite different. And some sequelae are so debilitating that the survivor can barely function.

Keep a journal

I encourage you to keep a journal, every day if possible. Your main purpose is to note important developments related specifically to your injury. This is good for you to know, but also for your caregiver and recovery team. Your doctors and therapists will all ask you "how have you been?" and your journal will help you share honestly and specifically what your day-to-day life is like.

Part 1: Everyday Events

When I began keeping one, my first challenge was just to remember what I had eaten the previous day. I wrote it all down just to test my memory, which helped me frame the rest of the day so I could jot down what I had done besides eat. So in the beginning, your journal will not be all that interesting. You are simply trying to re-capture the events of the previous day.

Part 2: Significant Injury-Related Events

Also note major injury-related events, such as:

- Cognitive exertions (conversation, sorting laundry, whatever is a cognitive exertion for you), and how long you did them

- Physical or emotional repercussions of those exertions (dizziness, extreme fatigue, disfluency, stuttering, headaches)

- Time and duration of rest periods; distinguish between simple rest and actual sleeping

- Important conclusions you can draw from the exertion/repercussion cycle; for example, if you notice that you have an especially rough day after seeing a movie the night before, you might decide that a movie theater is not a good environment for you.

Sequelae and everyday life

Shortly after my injury I noticed that Lynne had underlined in a brochure the disabilities she recognized in me (see below). "Brain Injury: The Multiple Disability," put out by the Massachusetts Brain Injury Association, states that the disabilities common to mild and moderate TBI fall into the following categories:

- **Medical**: seizures, headaches, dizziness, weakness of one or both sides, <u>fatigue</u>.

- **Sensory-Motor**: impaired coordination, <u>balance</u>, <u>speech</u>, <u>hearing</u>, sensation and <u>visual</u> problems

- **Intellectual-Cognitive**: <u>impaired attention and concentration, impaired reasoning, impaired memory, slowness of thought processes, difficulty reading and writing</u>

- **Social-Personality**: <u>agitation</u>, <u>emotional instability</u>, inappropriate social behavior

Any of these disabilities can hobble the daily life of a mild TBI survivor.

Sequelae make it hard to perform even these everyday activities:

- Attending a parent-teacher conference;

- Working out in a gym inundated with loud music, bright fluorescent lights, and the possibility of small talk and forced friendliness;

- Shopping for groceries;

- Walking through a mall;

- Dining out in a restaurant surrounded by music, background conversation and clanking of dishes and silverware.

As the following anecdotes show, even simple tasks can be really hard.

Organizing personal effects

One Saturday, Lynne cleared out clutter from our basement that had accumulated for years, and presented me with two boxes of my stuff. She asked me to go through it and decide what to keep and what to toss. Something that would have taken any normal person maybe 20 minutes took me an hour and a half, after which I promptly had to "shut down" to recover.

I've noticed that my tinnitus intensifies after any kind of extended cognitive exertion, so for me it's my red flag of warning. That loud ringing is a clear signal that I am overextending myself and need to stop whatever I'm doing.

A stack of miscellaneous papers taunt me. I have to look away because I see a hundred categories, and trying to sort it all would mean analyzing and decision-making, which quickly saps my cognitive energy. Imagine a cell phone just sitting on your desk. The battery bars don't move much, but if you start using it, the bars start disappearing.

That's why it's hard to bring order to the coffee table, sort through the surface clutter on my bureau and desk, sort laundry, clean the kitchen, clean out the interior of my car, and pay bills. But I do all of these things. They are all part of everyday living, and worth the cost.

TBI survivors eventually learn that most of life is draining. While we have to weigh whether doing a particular thing is worth the aftermath, we can't always offer a flat "no" to the people we care about, and sometimes even this deliberation is exhausting. If the kitchen is a mess, more often than not the right thing to do is to put the dishes in the dishwasher, empty it and put all the dishes away. That simple act might make us lie down for an hour afterwards, but at least we will feel useful and lighten the load of others.

Using a computer and using the internet

Many TBI survivors find the sheer physical act of staring into a computer screen difficult, especially with older models. A damaged brain does not do well with images that vibrate and flutter even slightly, and concentration is almost impossible. (It took a support-group meeting two years later to find out that wearing blue glasses helps.) Add to that the difficulty of sorting through e-mails, deciding which to answer when and how thoroughly. I often fantasize about getting off the Internet entirely, but sheer loneliness keeps me connected.

At the same time, this technology can offer meaningful tools if we know how to use them to our advantage. Facebook in particular has been a real boon to my feeling of community and refreshing old friendships that I'd forgotten were meaningful and pleasurable. And I handle e-mail in manageable parts now, a few at a time.

Following a recipe

I didn't do a lot of cooking before the injury but I could certainly follow a recipe – something I now find really hard to do. Obviously, this task requires an ability to sequence, interpret and customize information. Let's say we're having six people over for dinner and the recipe is for four. The simple arithmetic required to adapt it for six makes following the recipe even more difficult, especially under the time pressure of our guests' arrival. Even having to choose a recipe is challenging because it means evaluating what food we already have, what food I have to shop for, and where I have to shop for it.

So when we have guests over now, the best bargain is to let Lynne do all of that, and I clean up the next morning. We each play to our strengths. Chapter 22 is all about these kinds of strategies for couples.

Reading

Early on, I found I could read only a page or so of substantial writing, which told me something about my limitations. What I didn't know was whether that would improve over time, or if entire realms of literature were now closed to me.

Something about the newspaper felt just about right. I could browse a wide variety of articles, land on something that caught my eye, and most of the pieces that interested me were short. I often found that I would forget what was in the paragraph I'd just read and have to go back and re-read it, but that level of comprehension improved over time.

One time, Gregg told me something very basic but it stuck with me. I was reading a novel in the middle of the day, and after just an hour of what I considered light reading, I felt absolutely wiped out. We talked on the phone and I said, "Most people would love to have a day just to read a novel. Why can't I even enjoy that?" Gregg said, "John, we're not like most people."

Making travel arrangements

I have a hard time deciphering train schedules for my trips to and from Boston, but that problem pales in comparison to my costly travel arrangement errors. One such mistake cost Lynne and me a night at a hotel in the San Francisco airport. We ended up taking a later flight, but at great expense.

I struggle with travel arrangements because it's hard to:

- Figure costs in relation to our budget

- Identify the best travel times because of airline blackout dates in relation to Lynne's work schedule

- Work with a travel agent or use Internet travel sites to purchase tickets

- Choose one hotel or restaurant or activity over another

- Plan ground transportation

- Go over my decisions with Lynne

Evenings with friends

I've spent wonderful and hilarious evenings with a limited number of friends and my injury has been pretty invisible. The next morning Lynne might say, "You did really well last night!" and she'd be right. But I always feel compelled to remind her what we talked about: easy, relaxed, uncomplicated things like baseball, movies or music. And after those fun evenings I generally paid a heavy price afterwards, feeling terribly and with amplified symptoms.

Not reading facial expressions or body language so well

After an outdoor barbeque with a bunch of people we didn't really know all that well, Lynne told me that one of the women had been flirting with me pretty outrageously. I remembered she had been nice to me, but from Lynne's vantage point, the woman's advances were pretty obvious, no doubt emboldened by her prodigious alcohol consumption that evening. Fortunately, both Lynne and I laughed about this.

Something we didn't laugh about was when we met with a lawyer who specializes in Social Security Disability Benefits. On the drive home I asked her, "Well, what did you think?"

"You couldn't tell?"

I said, "What do you mean?"

She said, "I thought he was so arrogant!"

It hadn't occurred to me to consider his arrogance because I knew he was handling something I couldn't. But this experience showed me that I had lost my ability to accurately read body language and facial expressions. I had no idea what Lynne had thought of him and, believe me, before the injury I would not have had to ask.

Time in a grocery store

At a presentation one evening a graduate student asked me, "How did you know you shouldn't spend more than 15 minutes in a grocery store?" Without weighing how it would sound, I blurted out, "Because I stood there wanting to be carried away on a stretcher with my face covered to hide the shame. Instead, I had to go to the checkout, load the bags into my car, drive home, and enlist help getting them into the house and putting them away." Well, the student wanted the truth, so I gave her the truth. If I had tried to be more tactful or image-conscious, I might have tried to sound less desperate.

Recycling at the dump

A few months into my recovery I felt well enough to go back to the dump with our garbage and recyclables on Saturdays. After a few Saturdays, however, I started figuring out why this was a supremely unpleasant and draining outing.

First of all, pawing through the various recyclables at home and then at the dump sapped me quickly and powerfully. The act of sorting felt like I was agitating a badly bruised part of my brain. Mentally going through all those categories of newspapers, magazines, plain paper, cardboard, plastic designated #1, and plastic designated with other numbers – under the time pressure of people waiting behind me – made me feel like a doddering old man. And every time a glass bottle crashed into the big metal recycling bin, the sound was so painful it felt like an explosion in my brain.

As if that were not enough to make us hire curbside trash pickup, I would also run into people I knew at the dump. They would ask, "How have you been?" To this day that question "floods" my brain and I have to work so hard to respond without stuttering and stammering that the effort leaves me physically depleted.

Serving as liturgist, more or less

One Sunday I served as liturgist, which in the Lutheran tradition means I put on a robe and guide the congregation through the service. Because this was a ceremonial day, in the narthex – the church's lobby – before service, our pastor explained that the four elders of the church would each carry one item down the aisle in procession: the cross, the Bible, a basin of water, a goblet of wine. We were one elder short so he asked that I carry the goblet of wine. He told us the order we were to walk in, and where to bow at the altar and then to turn left or right to our seats at the front of the sanctuary.

I neither followed nor retained his directions, which was embarrassing in front of the elders. One of them tried to clarify them for me but I still didn't get it. Our pastor further simplified the directions for me, and I thought I got it, but when I walked down the aisle I realized I didn't know whether to stop and bow before or after the baptistery. I chose one and turned for my seat. Standing there as the congregation sang, I also realized I didn't remember whether I had just carried the baptismal water or the goblet of wine.

A painter's math

After about a year into the injury we had to have our house painted. The painter explained the following to me:

> I will charge you $5,500 to paint your house. If I powerwash the front porch but don't stain it, I will reduce the price by $550. If I don't powerwash the front porch or stain it, I will reduce the price by $700.

I could not grasp this math. Lynne tried explaining it to me but I kept forgetting things in mid-conversation: "So we do or don't want him to powerwash the front porch?" I had to write down exactly what we wanted to tell the painter.

Handling mundane tasks

Lynne, of course, because she lives with me, notices the effects of my sequelae when I try to handle even the most mundane tasks:

> Tom, a friend of ours, called with the name of a notary. He knows about John's injury, and speaks clearly and deliberately with him. But

Tom still said the name too quickly for John to process it, nor could John even begin to write it down.

Tom repeated the name a second time and John managed to remember a few of the first letters. Tom repeated the name a third time, but this time John failed to remember the first few letters.

After the third attempt John said, "Tom, I can't do this." Tom said that he would e-mail the name. For a "normal" individual jotting down the name of someone would have been the simplest of transactions.

Lynne has made plenty of other observations:

We were at our youngest son's baseball game. John seemed to be feeling okay and he offered to get iced coffees. All he had to do was get in the car and drive to the store, but in the unfamiliar neighborhood he had to backtrack down a dead end street, and when he finally found the store it was closed.

He had to improvise by going to another store, but he got lost because of the effort involved in negotiating Saturday traffic. He had to ask for directions back to the baseball field but had trouble retaining them.

These two non-events made him feel so poorly that he was unable to watch the rest of the game. He remained in the car with his eyes closed and a towel over his face.

She adds a few more examples:

These deficits also make it hard for John to use vending machines (especially for purchasing tickets), piece together electronics or sports equipment, and decipher Post Office posters that describe the differences between Express Mail and Priority Mail.

In general, improvising or having to think on his feet is so much harder now, and any surprise – even something so simple as a newly posted Do Not Enter road sign – can throw him off and force him to use energy he needs to conserve.

As we've seen, whether in the first year of recovery or beyond, many people with mild TBI struggle to perform the simplest of tasks. And, as a result of the effort involved, TBI survivors can unravel emotionally and experience intense crash-and-recovery cycles. This of course affects our family members, and we often worry that our difficulties are undermining our relationships with them. That is the subject of Chapters 21, 22, and 23.

Why is answering open-ended questions so hard?

Let's look at another aspect of everyday life. Think of how much information you have to process when someone asks a simple question like, "How are you?":

- Is the person just making small talk?

- How much should I say?

- Saying I feel lousy sounds like I'm a pessimist and a loser, and I need to be more of a winner with a winning attitude towards life.

- If I just say, "Fine, thanks!" the person might think I've recovered.

- When was the last time I spoke with this person? Have I mentioned the latest breakthrough I made? Or the defeat that turned into a victory because I learned from my mistake?

- What if I've just gone through four terrible days in a row?

- When will I know if I've dominated the conversation and the person just wants to wrap it up?

- How do you ask, "and how are you?" without sounding like it's an afterthought, because after all, my recovery is the most interesting, pressing thing on my mind.

If you do not have a brain injury, you take a few seconds to marshal your cognitive energies and to process a huge amount of information, quickly differentiating between the likely intentions behind the question. If you have a brain injury, the possibilities for how to answer this question feel overwhelming and we are likely to just freeze.

And, if we have not been to a good Speech-Language Pathologist (SLP), we are likely to start stammering, buying time before attempting to get our act together and respond. One time when I started stammering in his office, my SLP, Rick Sanders, said something so simple that I was surprised I hadn't thought of it before. He said, "John, be sure you have thought through what you want to say before you try to say it." Of course! Rick elaborates:

> I often find that this kind of stuttering comes from diminished working memory and diminished sustained or selective attention. The person says his last sure word repeatedly while he attempts to reel in the rest of what he had intended to say, or find the words to make a point that has now become elusive.

Playing the brain injury card

Because I "present well," my cognitive difficulties are not immediately apparent. As I've heard in countless movies, desperate times call for desperate measures, and so sometimes you might have to play the brain injury card.

The first time was halfway through a very long day and I still had to get to Boston from the subway station. I was having trouble figuring out how to buy the new rail pass. Like an alcoholic who for the first time admits publicly he has a problem, I told a guy in a transit authority uniform, "I have a brain injury and I need help."

The second time I did this I was at the Wichita Airport after visiting my mother and my flight back to Boston had been cancelled. I looked around in kind of a stupor but that did not alert anybody to my need to find a nearby hotel for the night. I walked up to an airport employee in a red blazer and when I first explained my predicament he looked amused. I was just another harried traveler. Then I said, "I was in a car accident and I have a brain injury and I need your help." A switch flipped and he snapped into action, but in a very kind way.

The third time I played the brain injury card was visiting my father-in-law's rehab facility. Although it's only about 15 minutes away it took me 40 minutes the first time I drove there. I'd gotten lost, so by the time I got there I was feeling pretty disabled.

At the entrance the simple security instructions confused me: I pressed the wrong button and fumbled the numbers I was supposed to enter on the keypad. The receptionist came out, pointed to the instructions, and clearly annoyed said, "That's why there's a sign."

Her rudeness wounded me, almost to the point of tears. I leveled with her and said, "I'm recovering from a brain injury and everything is hard right now." Her tone changed, but I resented feeling compelled to tell her that. If the instructions had been clearer and if she had acted patiently and treated me kindly, I never would have had to swallow my pride like that and admit to my injury.

Like I said, there will be times when you should just come right out and say you need help because you have a brain injury. Most people will want to help you if they know why you are struggling.

THE FIRST ANNIVERSARY OF THE ACCIDENT

Using the D word

Just before the one-year anniversary of my car accident a number of things happened that forced me to use the word "disability" . . . and the word began to settle into my consciousness.

Both Rick, my Speech-Language Pathologist, and Sally, my social worker, warned me about how I might react to the first-year anniversary. They anticipated that I might revisit my loss and feel melancholy. But the day sort of came and went, and the family actually had a good evening together.

Andrew took us out for dinner at Outback, using a gift certificate his school gave him two years before at his eighth-grade graduation. That was the night Will went to the men's room after he ordered, and when his dinner came, Andrew jokingly brought it to him, still sitting in the stall.

That was also the night Andrew and I watched David Ortiz hit his 52nd homerun of the season, and when he got to the dugout all the players ignored him, giving him the silent treatment. Then they all burst out laughing, and started patting him and hugging him.

That was also the night Andrew had left notes for us on our pillows, telling us of his admiration for what both of us were enduring.

The day after the anniversary

The next day hit me pretty hard. I fed and watered the chickens in our backyard, growing sadder and sadder, and sat down on a bench by our pond. I went inside, checked some e-mails, and got even sadder and teary, and when I told Lynne what I was feeling, my words broke up and got tangled.

The previous two days had been very busy so this might have just been one of those let-down bad days, but whatever the reason I was in a really dark place.

Ever the go-getter, Lynne said, "Go swimming!" And I did, for a full 30 minutes, and I felt a lot better.

When I got back from the pool, though, I had what was for me a rather awkward moment with an elder from our church. We had hired him to do some handyman-type work around the house and he was on the front porch fixing a light. Up I walked holding my gym bag in the middle of the day, and we got to talking about a few church matters.

As you might imagine, this was a complex dynamic with many layers given that he was doing work on our house while I had been at the gym. I felt he might be thinking it was an indulgence for me to go to the gym, or that somehow I should know how to do the work he was doing, or that if I could go to the gym then I must be feeling pretty good. And all of this second guessing of what he might be thinking can unravel an already fraying state of mind.

While it's not good to dwell on or worry about appearances, if it's stressing you, then change the appearance. I got into work clothes and attacked the wild rose bushes and purple loosestrife taking over our property, which I found gratifying.

What not to say to a TBI survivor

The list of what not to say to a TBI survivor could be very long. Though usually meaning to convey concern, people can say the most unsettling and even painful things. I call these "show-stoppers" because conversationally they leave you dead in your tracks. A few that come to my mind are:

- "My son had eight concussions."

- "Did you have a relaxing day today, Mr. Byler?"

- "Put it behind you and move on."

- "You weren't this blunt before the injury."

You don't know where to begin to respond. And this paralysis quickly leads to the survivor's:

- sense of alienation from those around him, and loneliness

- confusion about what is happening to him

- creeping depression

Better not to say much

I think the best advice I can give visitors is that talking is over-rated. One woman I know was in very rough shape in the first weeks of her injury. She said the best visit she got was her real-estate agent, who didn't even know her very well. The lack of familiarity that limited their conversation was the very thing that improved the visit immeasurably. She came into my friend's room, sat down next to her, held her hand and barely said a word for 20 minutes; at which point she got up, leaned over and, kissing the top of her head, smiled and said goodbye.

Both relative silence (and the silence of relatives) and these simple expressions of affection are so needed by the brain injured. We know we don't communicate well anymore – whether the listening or the talking – and, because we often find it hard to read body language and facial expressions, a hug and an arm squeeze and perhaps a kiss on cheek do wonders not found in most texts of higher learning.

Also welcome, if genuine, are expressing respect for our strength, our poise, our courage throughout this adversity. Assure us that you will be thinking of us often, and will call ahead of time if you plan to visit. A card, even two months into our recovery, will be of some comfort and strength.

So again, stillness is a virtue. Keep the visit very low key. Just your presence says, "I'm here for you." Try to make your facial expressions sort of obvious and your voice in the lower registers. Don't laugh sharply, loudly, or too frequently. Even if outdoors, use your indoor voice. And finally, be very aware of the time. A visit with a brain injury patient should be brief, something like 20 to 30 minutes tops.

Adding insult to Elizabeth's injury

Elizabeth e-mailed me after seeing my video, and we started quite a correspondence. After we spoke for an hour on the phone I knew we would comprise another two-person support group, along with me and Gregg, and me and Mike. Elizabeth sent me this list of showstoppers she drew up just to get it out of her system, and I can tell you that this list is common among survivors:

- "The damage to the car wasn't that bad." – *Dad*

- "You've never had this much on your mind." – Mom (after telling her about how I hallucinate when my headaches get really bad)

- "You are a beautiful girl! Why would you behave this way?" – *Co-worker*

- "You have Post-Traumatic Stress Syndrome." – *ER doctor*

- "You have a little girl . . . You really need to get better." – *Co-worker*

- "You don't have a brain injury. You have something else that I'm not qualified to discuss." – *Neuropsych evaluator*

- "You're not dying!" – *Co-worker*

- "If your symptoms are acute, you need to just go to the hospital." – *Supervisor*

- "You're not talking like somebody with a brain injury." – *Lawyer*

- "You're never going to find a doctor who can tell you what this is." – *Primary Care Physician*

- "These drawings are what I would see in-patient schizophrenics do." – *Psychologist*

Lifelines of humor

After a friend of ours saw the video on YouTube she said, "I liked it but do you think it was appropriate to have so much humor in it, given the seriousness of the topic?" I explained that if she ever went with me to a support-group meeting she would see that survivors look for every opportunity to laugh. We spend so much of any given day feeling awful, and so it is unusually refreshing for us to laugh.

One morning, about a year after the accident, I woke up in bed and, for the first time in my recovery, I started composing a parody in my head. This would not have been unusual in my pre-injury days. That morning I kept thinking of new phrases and sentences, and I started feeling the familiar excited surge of adrenaline in my body and some wonderful chemical in my brain that I hadn't felt in a year. I knew I had to get up and start writing before I forgot it. Here's pretty much what I wrote that morning:

> Dear Kind Sir Mr JOHN BYLER
>
> Please me allow introduce self. I am the deposed king of a small, obscure country and after years of very benevolently ruling my beloved country with an iron fist I was unceremoniously given my walking papers in what was fortunately for me a bloodless coup. I'd always told my late father Henri before he reached his untimely end that if I had to go in a coup, please might it be a bloodless one.
>
> The thing of it is I seem to have left some serious gold bullion in a shoe box hidden on a high shelf in my royal closet and I think it best to try and retrieve it before it gets in the hands of less enlightened and ruling class folk who in your country you call common rabble. It would perturb me greatly if this were to happen. You can only imagine my perturbation.
>
> Where do you come in, you might be wondering, Mr JOHN BYLER? Well I'm glad you asked because if you could see your way clear to sending me via wire or check or Paypal the sum of $800 – which I will repay with unbelievable interest in three months – you will enable me to take skydiving lessons upon completion of which I will enact a cunning plan involving a parachute, helmet and goggles.

Now that I think of it if you could also send an additional $100 I could purchase a pair of shoes I've had my eye on. They have giant and powerful springs because there is the matter of the rather formidable wall over which I must jump not once but twice, the second time as I make my exit, hopefully without detection of said rabble.

My memories of my glory and salad days are but memories. I long to return to my court, where the royal we would spend many hours surrounded by our formerly faithful armed militia, feasting and cavorting after hard fought coup quelling, laughing to the antics of my jester Lars.

Who are you Mr JOHN BYLER to say that this is not as things should be always? Please at your earliest convenience remit to me a loan of $900 and you will rejoice in my happiness and share in my mutinous bounty.

Sincerely, the former King Henri Jr.

I was thrilled. This too was awareness because I was becoming aware not only of my limitations. I saw that I had not lost my sense of humor, and an important part of my life – creativity, satire – was slowly being restored.

In this section on Awareness you've seen how I and three other survivors were "knocked into another dimension," and then how my first week, month and year unfolded. It became painfully clear that one of our biggest frustrations early in our recovery was the lack of a proper diagnosis. After reading about my new friend David's misdiagnosis, we'll look closely at some of the factors that contribute to misdiagnosing TBI, particularly the "mild" variety.

6 – Misdiagnosis Case Study: David

DAVID HITS HIS HEAD

"They all just blew me off, and that was a terrible thing to do."

Getting a brain injury in a library "for God's sake!"

Another new friend David danced with American Ballet Theater when famed dance impresario Lincoln Kirstein saw his intellectual potential and encouraged him to go to college after his dance career ended. David took Kirstein's advice, and after teaching dance in Munich, Germany he studied at UC Berkeley where he earned a degree in information and library science. The university hired him to work in Special Collections where David was working when he injured his brain:

> In Special Collections you're always on top of one another in a small space, and I was working on the floor when somebody I knew pulled out a drawer above my head. I remember that it was exactly 12 noon when I stood up and hit the back of my head very hard on that bony protuberance at the base of your skull. Doctors said it was probably the best place to hit it because the protuberance protects the brain.

He saw a GP at the university medical center immediately after the accident. She gave him the "infamous neurological test, the silly one where they ask you to name the last six presidents of the U.S. or count back from 100 by 7," and when David managed to perform to her expectations, she released him. He went home, put an ice pack on his head to alleviate a throbbing headache, and reassured himself: *"Of course you have a headache; you hit your head."* He figured that his symptoms were normal for the first 24 hours after the injury, and assumed he would be okay – as have so many of us who ended up with mild TBI.

After several days he noticed a "buzz" in his head. Then, because his intense headache persisted, he saw his primary care physician who told him, "You hit your head; it will take time to get better." He handed David off to a worker's compensation neurologist who saw David every month for a period of six months. No problems ever showed up on David's MRI, so the neurologist, unable to do anything for him, simply told him – repeatedly – that he was going to be fine.

David sustained his injury more than 15 years ago, but many doctors continue to be dismissive of patients seeking treatment after a "mild" head injury. The Web site for Mt. Sinai, a venerable Manhattan institution at the cutting edge of mild TBI diagnostics and treatment, explains:

> Those who receive a blow to the head with brief (or no) loss of consciousness are often sent home from the hospital with assurances that they are just fine. However, this may or may not be the case, and when not the case, this misinformation about no long-term problems may have devastating effects, as the person remains unaware of the basis for his or her altered ability to function.

After seeing my video on YouTube David got in touch with me and said:

> If my doctors had told me everything that I know now, I would have "healed" more quickly. What I mean by that is my anxiety would have been less; I would have put up with my sequelae much better; I would have had less fear; and that is the word that says it all: "fear". I was very fearful that I had damaged myself permanently and no doctor allayed my fears. They all just blew me off and that was a terrible thing to do.

"You should be all right by now"

"The people with mild TBI are the ones who are frustrated frustrated frustrated. And we get so desperate." David

"Talk about frustrating!" David says of doctors who failed to take his injury seriously:

> My headaches went away, but I wasn't the same. I had ongoing problems beyond what the doctor said I should have had, and he kept saying, "You should be all right by now." So I demanded to go to the hospital where I was given another MRI. The hospital neurologist said, "It's clean," and I said to her, "I've heard that before."
>
> She asked me, "How long have you been reading your book?" – she was referring to a book I had with me – "Did you understand it?" When I said yes, she said, "You're gonna be just fine," and I can't begin to tell you how I felt when she just turned on her heel and walked out of room. So I got no help from anybody.
>
> I was blown off by all the doctors. It was all about "you didn't lose consciousness" and "you're gonna be fine." I was in San Francisco and in New York City and saw the most sophisticated people and didn't get the help I needed.

DAVID BEGINS TO RESEARCH TBI

Comparing the current state of research to AIDS research in the 1980s

While he was working at Berkeley as a librarian in the 1990s, David did a lot of epidemiological research on AIDS. It was his impression that mild TBI was as misunderstood in the 1990s and today as the scourge of AIDS was in the 1980s.

His impression still has validity, and it is certainly reinforced by the barrage of media attention to the devastating effects of under-diagnosed or misdiagnosed head injuries sustained in football, soccer and other sports – consider the widely publicized death of actress Natasha Richardson who fell while skiing on a gentle slope – and in the wars in Iraq and Afghanistan. The media buzz is contributing to a growing public awareness that medical professionals need to look more closely at "mild" head injury.

The "second wave"

David had come to think that "where you hit your head and how hard you hit it" had to be critically important factors in a TBI – a reasonable theory – but "nobody, not one of my doctors, ever asked me, 'Where were you hit? How hard were you hit?'" A phenomenon called the "second wave" – also called Second Impact Syndrome – intrigued him:

> About 48 hours after an injury, chemicals enter into the brain, and the effects can be very disconcerting. I thought I was simply feeling the impact but…it was the release of chemicals into the brain that was making me feel as I did. The thing is, with most people who have a mild injury, you're discharged, and this "second wave" happens after you're discharged. So there are a lot of questions about the effect of these chemicals.

TBI scales

As of this writing, there is still no standard TBI scale universally accepted throughout the medical community that effectively distinguishes mild from moderate and severe TBI. Doctors use a variety of scales, and some scales are more widely used than others, but the lack of a single standard scale points to the fact that clinicians have yet to develop a full understanding of how to diagnose mild TBI. All you have to do is Google "TBI scales" to get a sense of how many are out there and the extent to which they overlap.

What does appear to be standardized is the almost knee-jerk clinical response to a patient who goes to an emergency room or a neurologist's office with a head injury. David recalls:

> Every doctor I saw asked me if I had lost consciousness and when I replied in the negative, they immediately blew me off. The consciousness/
> unconsciousness thing seems to be a gate. The moment you say no, you didn't lose consciousness, they lose interest . . .
>
> Once the MRI is clean, they really blow you off. Neurosurgeons, if they take a CT scan and find a blood clot, drill and do something, but when the CT scan and MRI are normal, for them, it's just "wait and see."

"We don't know . . ."

So we see that people with mild TBI can get pretty desperate and frustrated, but in one respect our desperation has been a good thing. It has forced us to find out all we can about mild TBI on our own. David devoted many months to researching mild TBI when doctors were unable to help him. He told me:

> You find out when you do research that it's like six degrees of separation. Every field has six to eight people who are state-of-the-art, and one person cites the other.

He came across the name of a state-of-the-art researcher of mild TBI in the Harvard Medical School journal and contacted him. The researcher turned out to be a Harvard-trained doctor at one of the country's leading research hospitals.

David asked this research doctor about damage to certain parts of the head: Does it matter which quadrant of the brain takes a blow? He also asked the researcher about the effect of the chemical releases: Are they harmful or helpful? Over a three-week period David asked him a lot of other questions as well, but the research doctor responded repeatedly, "Well, we don't know" and "People don't know."

David was persistent, but finally the researcher said to him, "Mr. B----, we just don't have answers to these questions."

The researcher's inability to answer his questions frustrated David, but I was actually somewhat reassured when David told me about these exchanges. So many doctors, especially neurologists, "think they know, but they don't" – a refrain I hear over and over from TBI'ers. In contrast, the Harvard researcher was bracingly, refreshingly, honest.

We don't know.

7 – Misdiagnosing "Mild" TBI

CHALLENGES OF DIAGNOSIS

"Can someone tell me what is happening to me?"

What really aggravates the first year of our recovery is that on top of feeling awful, our doctors, including neurologists, rarely say, "Everything you have experienced is consistent with a traumatic brain injury." We might hear this from other members of our team who work with TBI survivors all the time – Case Manager, speech pathologist, social worker – but many doctors don't come out and say it.

Five different neurologists might give five different diagnoses for the source of classic TBI symptoms. Three of the five might even say, "It's all in your head," which of course it is, but not in the way they think. What feels like doctors' dismissal of TBI symptoms intensifies our desperation. Survivors have so many questions and can't seem to find answers for any of them. I've drawn these examples from my own and other survivors' experiences:

- Why am I fatigued all the time?

- Why do I have to sleep so much? Or, why can't I sleep at all?

- What can I do about my dizziness, and these awful headaches?

- Why does the smallest task overwhelm me?

- Why can't I remember what I did yesterday?

- Why does dinner out with old friends torture me?

- Why do I feel so depressed?

- What do I say to people who are confused about my injury because I "look great?"

- Why can't I read much anymore, or figure out a train schedule, or balance my checkbook – and speaking of my checkbook, what do I do about my lost income?

- What do I say to my manager about all the work I've missed?

- Why is my spouse/partner so impatient with me? And so remote? Or am I misreading the situation . . . again?

- How do I deal with this crushing loneliness?

- Who can I turn to when I have suicidal thoughts?

Open question

Every survivor who is misdiagnosed has this question for the medical community:

> If doctors had been able to diagnose us quickly and correctly – or at the very least, if they had responded conservatively on the assumption that the cause of the symptoms was TBI – might our outcomes have been different?

These next two chapters do not call out by name any particular doctors I have seen. I assume that doctors want to help people with mild TBI – thank you, Hippocratic Oath. But as you will see, staggering amounts of evidence suggest that many doctors know little about it and often make misdiagnoses. As one BIAA Director told me:

> My experience working in the field and talking with people all over the country is that few neurologists really know anything about mild brain injury.

Recognizing symptoms of mild TBI

Brain injuries are among the most frequent reasons for physician and ER visits. The more you scratch the surface and talk with brain-injured people, the more you discover how few M.D.'s – even neurologists – recognize symptoms of so-called "mild" TBI, especially if an MRI and CT scan seem to indicate no physical damage to the brain.

In her review in *The New York Times* of the 2007 HBO special "Coma," Gina Bellafante states, "The uncertainty around severe brain injury, about which doctors still don't know a tremendous amount, seems unusually pervasive."[3] And this is much more the case when it comes to mild TBI, which is far more common and more subtle, but can still be devastating.

Second Impact Syndrome

As mentioned, I asked my Case Manager if I should have accepted the offer of an ambulance ride to the ER the night of my accident. She said that because I wasn't bleeding, I hadn't blacked out, and I could carry on a conversation, they would not have considered the possibility of a TBI. Consider Second Impact Syndrome, because doctors generally fail us on this:

> Second Impact Syndrome occurs when an individual experiences a second concussion less than two weeks after the first injury. This is extremely dangerous and can cause severe brain damage and death in some instances.[4]

I should not have gotten back into a car for at least two weeks after the accident – and athletes should not try and just shake off a concussion, or "wait till the cobwebs clear" before going back on the field. If a player *is* cleared to play the next game, and it is too soon, getting back on the field could be fatal, or at least cause permanent, more severe damage.

MY STORY MAPS A PATH COMMON TO MILD TBI SURVIVORS

Mild TBI narratives always begin with some sort of incident – a car accident, a fall, a stroke, brain surgery, the impact of a heavy object, even a severe sinus infection – followed by a medical response that is often grossly inadequate. Medical professionals, with all the good intentions in the world, send the survivor home with orders to "take it easy" and that's that. (This book, of course, hopes to give you more specific guidelines for recovery.)

Fear

The first aftershocks of the injury reverberate. The doctor is likely to dismiss or trivialize complaints, attributing them to anything but the incident. The survivor is scared. He (or she) has no idea what's wrong; all he knows is that he is not the same person that he was before the accident, and in many quantifiable ways.

Dr. Wayne Gordon, a highly regarded neuropsychologist with the Mount Sinai School of Medicine, has worked with thousands of TBI survivors for 40 years. He points out that the victim is often sent home and fails to connect his symptoms to the blows to the head he has sustained.[5] One after another harsh sequelae begin, and the fear makes it all worse. An early proper diagnosis can at the very least ease the fear because the survivor knows what is coming.

Misery

For weeks or months later, the aftershocks of the trauma, such as flu-like symptoms, memory loss, inability to concentrate, or crippling headaches and/or anxiety, are making the survivor miserable. He begins to seriously question his sanity because nobody has validated that what he is experiencing is real. It is also *normal* for someone who has sustained a brain injury.

He attempts to return to work, but can't perform up to par. He might seek assistance from his employer and begin to explore the benefits available to him through his employer's insurance, but his bosses and colleagues are unsympathetic, the insurance company becomes – or at least feels – adversarial, and it doesn't occur to him to contact an attorney. Meanwhile he sees another doctor (or series of doctors) who continue to misdiagnose him and label him with any number of maladies – except TBI, mild or otherwise.

Financial worries

Misdiagnosis is a consistent theme because knowledge about mild TBI is generally limited to the nation's top medical institutions, and often even doctors associated with these institutions misdiagnose. Ultimately the misdiagnoses are likely to make it difficult or impossible for the survivor to collect disability or health/treatment benefits without going to court.

If he decides to go to court, he will need a brain injury lawyer with real experience, and access to a team of expert witnesses on mild TBI. That's because the insurance companies and the employer might argue that the survivor's sequelae are not due to a brain injury, or is "malingering" – faking an injury. Insurance company witnesses might say something like, "It's not like he's paralyzed," which insurers have actually said to survivors I know.

Meanwhile, friends have dropped away and family members are at a loss. The survivor feels completely overwhelmed, and very, very alone.

Feelings of helplessness

Since 2005 when he had his accident, Gregg (Chapter 2) has been working together with his wife Diana to cope with his injury, which occurred on the day of their thirteenth wedding anniversary. During the year that followed, among Diana's greatest challenges was the helplessness she felt, as both a nurse and a wife.

The old saying is wrong: ignorance is <u>not</u> bliss

She and Gregg soon discovered the medical community's ignorance about how to diagnose and treat TBI:

> Gregg was so miserable. It was so desperate in the beginning, when we didn't understand the injury, and it was a year before he got into decent therapy. We struggled for a whole year.
>
> One of the hardest things we faced was that we had a lot of medical people pointing the finger at Gregg and saying, "It's psychological." That's baloney. For years they thought Lyme disease was psychological, and there was a time when they thought ulcers were psychological. Well, we know that Lyme and ulcers are real, physiological problems.
>
> As technology improves and more advances in research are made, at some point we'll be able to look at cellular responses and brain chemistry and be able to say with certainty "That's TBI" – and confirm that it, too, is a real physiological problem.

> But right now they want to be able to see it on a CT scan or on a slide and we're not there yet, although we can see the ravages of TBI on post-mortems now. Even the latest research is saying that TBI is "psychological" and that's wrong. We just don't have the tools to identify this injury with accuracy yet.

Being blown off: a theme

My new friend Elizabeth wrote to me:

> Problem is I've been blown off. These doctors either are too baffled and are ignorant to the injury . . . maybe hope I'll just go away and be somebody else's problem as they don't know what to do with me. Or they know it's worse than I realize and they don't want to tell me. How can I trust them now?

DOCTORS MUST LEARN TO LISTEN

. . . because we know something they don't

Our TBI strategy sessions in a major rehab hospital in New York City met three times a week for three months. Rose tended to hang back and not say much. She had injured her hand and brain in a mishap at a paper-manufacturing plant. One day the group leader asked us to talk about what triggered our most intense emotions. Rose opened up:

> Doctors are my trigger, especially neurologists who don't know what they're talking about, and dismiss what I have to say about my injury. I haven't had a satisfactory meeting with a neurologist yet. No neurologist has listened – really listened – to me talk about my injury without being patronizing, contemptuous and skeptical.

At this particular meeting three neuro-psychologists were helping us identify any distortions in our thinking. All three respectfully suggested to Rose that she look for possible flaws in her absolutist view of her doctors. Convinced that she was making a sweeping generalization that would fail to hold up under scrutiny, they then opened the question up to the group. They asked us, "Is Rose's thinking distorted?"

To their astonishment, every one of us agreed with Rose. I took notes on some of the survivor responses:

- "Every time I leave a neurologist's office, I'm angry and frustrated."

- "One of my neurologists wrote 'angry Latina" in his report. He attributed my sequelae to my ethnicity!"

- "I argued with my neurologist after I did some research on mild TBI, but he still didn't listen to me because they choose to learn more about it from journal articles than from the survivors sitting in front of them."

- "They think they know everything, but they're really in the dark about mild TBI."

- "The first neurologist I saw didn't even let me finish describing my sequelae. He interrupted me to say that my problems were due to the meds I'm on for my hand injury."

- "My GP said I didn't need to see a neurologist. She told me I was depressed and that I should see a shrink."

The three neuro-psychologists did persuade us to say with more precision "my doctor," instead of "all" doctors, but each of us insisted that we spoke the truth about our personal experiences.

But of those 85% . . .

Doctors give us statistics based on a timeline when we are first diagnosed with TBI; for example, that 85 percent of people with mild TBI return to work within one year. What they don't tell you, maybe because the data is too new, is that of the 85 percent who return to work, 80-85 percent believed they returned too soon.

In any case, those of us – and our numbers are legion – who do not recover within one year are made to feel as though we are statistical outliers. We don't represent the majority of cases. Isn't it foolish to ignore or discount a whopping 15 percent? (Fifteen percent of the estimated 1.7 million brain injuries a year in the U.S. comes to 255,000. If you subtract 52,000 deaths from TBI from 1.7 million, 15 percent of that is 247,200. Either way, an estimated quarter of a million people a year do not return to work in the first year of injury.)

It is not just a play on words to suggest that we outliers are made to feel like liars, slackers, or that we're deluded. For mild TBI survivors early in their recovery, hearing stories about the frustrations of other TBI'ers can actually come as a relief. It reduces some of the feelings of isolation and loneliness in being a statistical outlier. Survivors find comfort in this shared experience.

New survivors have probably seen so many different doctors who have insisted that they are "all right," or who have attributed their complaints to a cause other than a head injury, that they worry they are going crazy. Brain injury specialists at Mount Sinai Hospital observe:

> Often the individual with a mild TBI returns to his or her daily life after the injury with very little if any awareness that the head injury will have ramifications – short-lived probably, but perhaps long-term. To individuals in this [latter] situation, they notice out of the blue that in big and little ways they are no longer able to do what came easily before.

"For no reason that I can see, what I know about myself is no longer true." These inexplicable difficulties, which they do not associate with the "blow to my head," can lead the person to feel that he or she is losing it. [6]

"I haven't been handling this right for the last 35 years!"

Researchers assert that "as many as 80 percent of [mild TBI injuries] go undiagnosed" and that mild TBI is a "silent epidemic."[7] To be fair, many doctors do know that mild TBI can deal a severe blow, and some are crusading to inform their peers about it. Some doctors bravely admit that they have failed to diagnose mild TBI in the past.

"My jaw dropped open," one doctor confided when he learned that he had been misdiagnosing mild TBI for decades. "I'm looking at page after page [of notes on patients] and saying to myself, wow, I haven't been handling this right for the last 35 years."

FOLLOWING UP ON TOM

Misdiagnosis

Tom (Chapter 2) says this about his misdiagnosis:

> On my way to Boston [to] work I was hit head-on twice as my car spun around, with airbags deploying and the fourth vertebrae in my back smashed into pieces…Almost immediately after the accident I started to have some serious symptoms. Night sweats, panic attacks, mania, depression and other new and unwelcomed changes came every day.

> When I was no longer able to concentrate on my work as a banker and contacted my company's Employee Assistance Program, I was sent from doctor to doctor and told that…I now had mental illness.

Tom's difficulties had everything to do with the accident – the force of an impact strong enough to fracture his vertebrae was obviously strong enough to damage his brain. But Massachusetts' Employee Assistance Program (EAP) didn't see it that way. They sent Tom to a psychologist who diagnosed Tom with post-traumatic stress disorder (PTSD). "Nobody ever referred Tom to a neurologist," Arthur says, "and his primary care physician (PCP) brushed him off. We never had a chance to even consider another diagnosis."

Tom met next with a psychiatrist employed by the bank's insurance company. Like the psychologist, he never suggested that Tom's sequelae – the panic attacks, the night sweats, the inability to sleep, the sudden crying, the claustrophobia – were the result of his brain injury. Instead he attributed Tom's problems to his sexual preference:

> The doctor didn't write down a thing I told him about the accident and interrupted me to ask questions about my life before the accident. He asked me stuff about my being gay and about my relationship with my kids and my brother. He attributed my breakdown to my relationship with my brother, to my being gay and to my divorce from my wife. He did not attribute any of my difficulties to my accident and a traumatic brain injury. He dismissed it entirely.

Before the accident, Tom had no mental health problems. Now he wondered if he was losing his sanity. "So I meet with the psychiatrist and now I think I'm a mental case. Plus I can't go back to the work I loved. I've lost my life, and I feel useless. I labeled myself. I felt I could no longer be part of society. I was devastated."

Clearly, to the extent that a timely, accurate diagnosis can alleviate symptoms – or at least help a survivor anticipate and prepare for them – a misdiagnosis can similarly aggravate them.

Falling through the cracks of a broken system

The bank's employment handbook stated that the company would provide "rehabilitation and job coaching," but when Tom requested the assistance the bank refused on the grounds that Tom's problem were "psychiatric." Tom decided to seek workman's compensation, a step he probably should have taken immediately after the car accident given that commuting between branches was part of his job.

He contacted a lawyer, who encouraged Tom to get an MRI to determine the cause of his back and neck pain. (This is truly telling. Two years after his accident, after having seen a number of doctors, it took a neurolawyer to tell him to get an MRI!) Tom followed through and learned that he would need surgery to replace the smashed disc in his neck. After the surgery he completed his rehabilitation.

At that point the bank abruptly terminated all his health insurance benefits because the insurance company doctor had found nothing else wrong with him. The company standpoint was that Tom's problems were psychiatric. The psychiatrist urged Tom to get vocational rehabilitation, but the bank and the insurance carrier denied him coverage.

"You know, my anxiety started immediately after the accident," Tom recalls. "Feeling that level of anxiety and not knowing what it was probably worsened my panic attacks. I wish there had been a booklet in the emergency room that could have told me what I had. And medical people never really tested me. I had more in-depth tests when I had a kidney stone attack."

Insurers can feel adversarial

One of the worst things for Tom was that representatives of the insurance company questioned his integrity. Tom met with one to discuss his problems and "numerous times" the representative implied that Tom was lying about his condition. "It's not like you got your eye poked out," the rep said. "If you had a physical injury we would believe you, but you're telling us you have a psychiatric injury and we can't tell." Besides the fact that TBI is not a psychiatric injury, the representative's insinuation that Tom was lying contributed to Tom's apprehension about his mental health.

Meanwhile, he had discovered that long solitary walks in the natural world made him feel better. One day, though, he emerged from a hiking trail to see the insurer's van in the parking lot. Tom thought, "Oh my God, they're following me." From that day on he began to live in real and substantiated fear that the insurance company was spying on him:

> It made me paranoid. So after that I isolated myself.
>
> It got to the point where I was afraid to leave my house. Every time the doorbell rang or the phone rang, I was afraid it was the company and they were watching me. I'm not scamming them, but because I didn't get my eye poked out, they think I'm scamming them.

By the way, paranoia may well have set in with Tom, but insurers often do send field reps out to trail the insured. One rep sat with me for two hours having me restate my condition, and then played videotape of me in a grocery store for ten minutes. I had been followed from my driveway all the way to Spaulding Rehab in Boston, 35 miles away. That is all perfectly legal, but unsettling. The videotape even included me walking out of Spaulding, going to my car, stopping briefly at another car and taking a picture of the bumper. When the rep asked me why I'd done that, I explained that the bumper had stickers supporting both the Yankees and Red Sox, a rare sight in these parts.

Maybe this is not even necessary to say, but always tell the truth about every aspect of your injury and so-called recovery, and you need not live in fear of being watched.

SO-CALLED "MILD" TBI

"People can sustain a mild TBI and have traumatic outcomes." David

The word "mild"

When you're finally diagnosed with mild TBI your first thought is, "What do you mean, mild? Mild compared to what?" The first time I walked into Spaulding I saw "compared to what." My brain injury was mild compared to the severely brain injured people I saw in wheelchairs, or if they were even less fortunate, in rolling beds. Still, mild TBI was a catastrophe for me, and it turned my family, career and life upside down.

Following his accident in the UC Berkeley library, David (Chapter 6), a researcher by professional training, thoroughly investigated TBI. As he discovered, "mild TBI" is actually a clinical term: Doctors use "mild TBI" to refer to head injuries where there is no loss of consciousness. ("LOC" is the commonly used medical acronym for "loss of consciousness.")

Mild TBI: a "distinct clinical entity" that can be "inestimably costly"

Dr. Elaine Woo, former Program Director of the Spaulding Head Injury Program, recognizes that mild TBI is not minor. It is:

> a distinct clinical entity with its own unique problems to the patient…[and] a multifaceted syndrome. Despite apparently normal test results, many patients with mild head injury experience an array of symptoms spanning physical, cognitive and psychological functioning.
>
> [These include] a generalized impairment of all intellectual functions…but problems with memory, concentration and attention, judgment and abstract thinking are most prevalent.
>
> A residual unique to mild head injury is the problem of impaired quantitative intellectual functioning, which refers to the inability to process information successfully if speed or complexity is required.
>
> [The aftermath of mild TBI can] lead to life disruption and lost productivity…inestimably costly to the individual, his family and his community.

My SLP Rick Sanders discussed Dr. Woo's article with me, and said that she includes some patient quotes "that could come straight from you: 'They told me I would be okay,' 'My tests are normal,' 'There's nothing on the MRI,' 'Am I going crazy?'"

Not-so-mild sequelae

In strictly clinical terms doctors decided that David and I suffered "mild" TBIs simply because we didn't lose consciousness after our accidents. But – and this is huge – people with mild TBI do not necessarily have mild sequelae. Sequelae – the aftershocks or secondary effects of a brain injury – can disable a survivor for months, and even years, after a trauma.

"My worker's comp doctor just assumed my sequelae would go away," David says, but many people with mild TBI endure sequelae that handicap them for the rest of their lives. He adds, "What has to be really clear is that your life can be totally down the drain because of the sequelae. People can sustain a mild TBI and have traumatic outcomes." Experts at Mount Sinai agree:

> Although the negative consequences of mild TBI tend to disappear more or less quickly for most people who have mild injuries, some research suggests that about 15 percent continue to suffer symptoms that can be severely debilitating. Thus, "mild" injury may be anything but mild. *(Mount Sinai Hospital website)*

BRIEF COMMENT ON THE STATE OF "MILD" TBI RESEARCH

"Why is it that we patients have to do the identification, the research, the diagnosis, the prognosis?" David

Notes from the mild TBI underground

My personal experiences and the anecdotal reports of a lot of other people with mild TBI have convinced me that neurologists prefer to treat people they believe they can actually help, such as people recovering from stroke, or who have MS, Parkinson's or other degenerative diseases.

Rick Sanders clarifies this point:

> Although it is true that medications can greatly help these patients, those with degenerative diseases like MS and Parkinson's often succumb to their illnesses. So perhaps it is more the case that

> persistent symptoms from MTBI are not well understood...or we could say there is not a consensus on how to treat MTBI.

Maybe we shouldn't blame them. We all like to see positive results from the work we do. Because they know so little about mild TBI and it's not a degenerative disease, or as far as I know an affliction that directly kills people, they stand by and hope the patient will improve over time, letting "nature take its course."

You would think that of all people, neurologists could be counted on to stay current with neurological issues, but there were times when I wondered when they were going to apply the leeches. I am not the only one who feels this way. Aside from countless vent sessions in TBI support groups, a good friend of mine says this about her husband, who has suffered from brain-damaging seizures for years:

> You are so right about neurologists! Michael's first neurologist REFUSED to let me attend the sessions that were to establish what was causing blank spots in his memory. How much sense does that make? Neurological disturbances mean that you can't remember or don't recognize what you have forgotten. It would seem to me that an outside observer is crucial.

Considerable evidence suggests that the most up-to-date knowledge about mild TBI has failed to trickle down to – or "bubble up to" – neurologists, even at major hospitals. If this is true for the Boston area, home to many great hospitals, imagine the bleak prospects elsewhere.

Neurologists may well diagnose you with anything *but* mild TBI, such as depression, anxiety, stress, dementia, early onset Alzheimer's and even mental illness. However, you should contact a neurologist because, even if they attribute your problems to something other than mild TBI, they are highly trained to treat aspects of your suffering, such as intense headache and atypical migraines, balance issues and cognitive problems involving memory, language and speech.

8 – "Look, I'm not Phineas Gage!"

THE DOCTOR/PATIENT INTERACTION

". . . he was the very model of the couldn't-care-less doctor: arrogant, brusque, sarcastic." Jean-Dominique Bauby

Jean-Dominique Bauby, a French journalist paralyzed after a stroke, communicated by blinking one eye, and in fact dictated the entire book *The Diving Bell and the Butterfly* in this fashion. Although we do not have what is called "locked-in syndrome," I and many other TBI survivors can relate to much of what Bauby experienced. He notes, for one thing, "the veiled mistrust the medical profession always arouses in long-term patients."

The book also struck my SLP Rick Sanders:

> Bauby also writes eloquently about what it is like to be misunderstood…and about people who can't take the time to be with someone who processes or responds more slowly. I am particularly fond of his recounting of the time he was watching the Munich soccer game and the night nurse or some such person came in and asked him something perfunctory and without waiting for a response simply turned the television off – end of story.

As I went from doctor to doctor *I* knew that I was experiencing a new reality. Here were highly trained doctors, the supposed experts, insinuating that my sequelae were not due to the car accident. For a long time I didn't know anything about mild TBI so I couldn't push back with data other than my own experience. All I knew was that something bad had happened to me and I was feeling as though I was living inside a Kafka horror story.

The big question that survivors want to ask is, why do so few doctors seem to understand mild TBI?

Diffuse axonal injury

As I waited in the hospital cafeteria before seeing one doctor I noticed a hand-made poster created for visiting junior high-school students. In simple language, it described the difference between "focused" and "diffuse" axonal injury. I choked up because the description of the latter matched the circumstances of my accident exactly, and the stretching and tearing was consistent with the unfolding symptoms of my injury in the days that followed:

> . . . sudden slowing down from a high speed as in a car accident . . . nerves in the brain get stretched, causing them not to work correctly, swell and eventually separate. They do not usually rip at the time of the accident, but after hours or days.

I wrote the words in my journal in case the doctor I was about to see did not know what to make of me.

The moment I walked into his office, this doctor looked at me with what looked like a grave, let's-get-real expression. He immediately said he couldn't see anything on the new MRI he had evaluated. I knew how to read between the lines: If there was no evidence of an injury on an MRI, he felt entitled to conclude that I had no injury at all – a view that apparently still prevails among many doctors who routinely misdiagnose mild TBI.

I began to read to him from the notes I had taken on the poster, but he interrupted me and said, "I know all about diffuse axonal injury." I was so frustrated that I almost cried. Here I was at one of the leading brain injury centers in the country and the doctor was still focusing on the lack of evidence on an MRI. In effect, despite the overwhelming evidence of my sequelae, it felt as though he was dismissing me *and* my injury.

Now, of course, I frequently read articles that explicitly state what the poster was alluding to:

> The most common form of TBI is diffuse axonal injury, which interrupts communication between neurons. In concussion, a mild form of diffuse axonal injury, "the injured areas are usually so small, although spread out in many areas, that they do not show up on the usual brain scans such as CT, X-ray and MRI" . . . [8]

Our meeting rapidly degenerated. "Look," I said, "I'm not Phineas Gage!" (Gage, a complete medical anomaly, walked and talked after a huge railroad spike drove all the way through his skull in an accident back in 1848.) I explained that, first of all, I acknowledge that my brain injury is not of the severe variety. A railroad spike came nowhere near my brain's soft tissue.

But I also meant that Gage was just about a medical and statistical impossibility. I'm *not* one in a million. There are lots of people whose mild TBI is affecting them in very serious ways. I've met many of them and, most of all, I'm living with the results. (At one recent support-group meeting, we actually ran out of chairs. As I stood in the back of the room, looking around at all the new faces, I felt as though I was part of some kind of powerful grassroots movement.)

Figure 2:

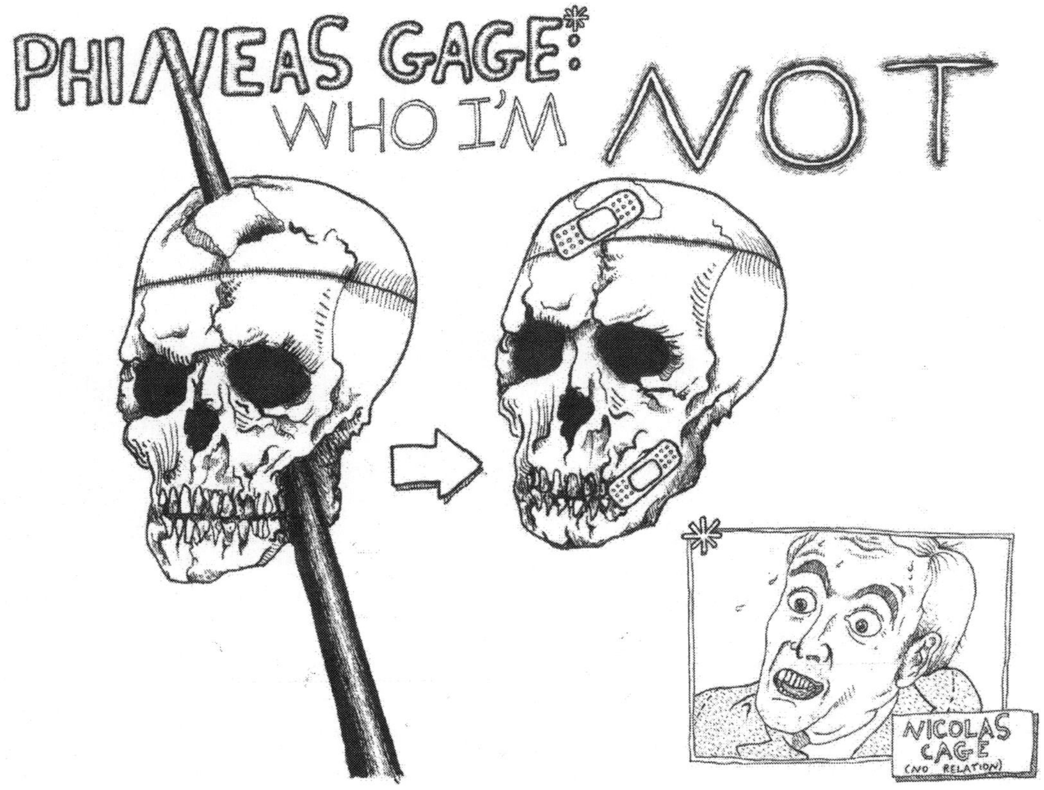

<u>*Artwork*</u>: *Chris Byler*

Still stunned, I reiterated my sequelae and told him that I believed it was due to the diffuse axonal injury I'd sustained in the car accident. In my mind, I felt I had connected the dots. All I wanted was for him to see the picture the dots created.

He looked at me with an expression my injured brain was unable to decipher and said, "You're obsessing over what happened the night of the accident." Irritated, I said, "I'm not obsessing about that night. I'm talking to you about it because you're my doctor." I thought, "What? Why are you changing the subject? Why won't you listen to me? I know something you don't – my own injury!" I told him I simply wanted to discuss treatment for the very real sequelae of my injury.

At the end of the meeting I said:

> You seem to be used to working with more severe cases of TBI, and so when someone like me comes into your office you might be thinking, "What's he worried about? At least he's walking around." Well, the truth is that I and many people with mild TBI are the walking wounded.

MY OWN MISDIAGNOSIS

Complying scrupulously with "Dr. X"

Determined to recover fully from my brain injury, I worked closely for almost three years with a well-regarded doctor – let's call him Dr. X. I took my interactions with each member of my recovery team so seriously that I dressed like I was going to a business meeting whenever I went to the hospital. I had decided that getting well was my new full time job, and I dressed for success.

Ritalin vs. Concerta

I was so desperate to feel better that I slogged through disastrous courses of medications. Dr. X started me with Namenda, normally prescribed for Alzheimer's patients, and as I ramped up all of my sequelae grew worse. Next, he prescribed the psychostimulants Ritalin and then Concerta, both of them categorized as Methylphenidate.

In retrospect, it disturbs me that prescribing increasing doses of Ritalin and then Concerta – 54 mg in the morning, and 36 mg at noon – was largely due to my simply requesting them. I do not recall him cautioning me that speeding an injured brain might not be conducive to healing. I felt as though I was numbing a broken arm with painkillers and then painting a ceiling all day.

Several years later, after swearing off any stimulants, including tea and coffee, I agreed to dip my toe in the ocean of Methylphenidate and today I have struck a very good balance: 5 mg of Ritalin in the morning, crashing hard for two hours after it has left my system, and then either 5 or 10 mg in the afternoon to see me through the rest of the day. For me, Ritalin works better than Concerta because the latter is time-release and so it never gave my brain an opportunity to rest, whereas Ritalin leaves the system after 4 or 6 hours.

Continuing with my so-called recovery

Anyway, I scrupulously complied with every one of his protocols, and at every meeting shared with him the misery of my day-to-day life. No brain damage showed up on any of the MRIs, fMRIs, CT scans and EEGs because, as anybody with mild TBI should know, none of these increasingly outdated technologies are sophisticated enough to record the stretching and tearing that can occur at the neuronal level as a result of a trauma. Despite all my efforts, efforts that my friends and family told me were "heroic," it became increasingly clear that my sequelae were getting worse and my "crash and recovery" cycles more intense and of longer duration.

I felt so badly that I was finally forced to recognize the probability that I would be unable to return to my livelihood. On the advice of several people, I applied for the continuation of my Long Term Disability (LTD) benefits. I laboriously cataloged my intensifying sequelae with Dr. X and the other members of my recovery team so the former could report to my insurance company.

A trauma to the doctor/patient relationship

To my astonishment, after years of working with me, and after confiding to him the darkness and misery of my new life, in his official report to my insurer Dr. X attributed literally 99 percent of my problems to sleep apnea – a mild annoyance that I had before the accident and is now under control – and depression. Needless to say, this did not help my case with the insurer, which already set strict new criteria after 24 months of injury.

David had a similar experience when his worker's compensation ran out and it was time for him to return to work.

> What was so upsetting to me was that my neurologist wrote, 'He has recovered fully,' and I hadn't. I had to file suit, and I won.

I am not a combative person, but I wrote a strongly worded e-mail to Dr. X. (A phone conversation would have been impossible.) He responded, expressing his confidence in his diagnosis based on "the consensus in the field":

> . . . people with mild TBI's generally recover, and if after 2 1/2 years you have not, there are likely other factors perpetuating your symptoms. I brought in the issue of psychological factors (not necessarily depression) and encouraged you to explore CBT [cognitive behavioral therapy]. This does represent a change in my perspective to some degree as the consensus in the field has turned in this direction (based on many studies), but also a matter of timing (the length of time since the injury).

What I wanted to say to him was, "Don't believe everything you read, doc. Sometimes you have to believe the patient sitting in front of you." He made his decision because of the "length of time since the injury." This is something many survivors hear, things like, "Frankly, I'm discouraged at your progress" and "Most people would be better by now!" Doctors can make survivors feel as though it is somehow their fault that they have not recovered.

Other members of my recovery team expressed different points of view from that of Dr. X. One person wrote to me very tactfully:

> My perspective is that persons who experience an acceleration-deceleration injury have likely incurred diffuse axonal injury which affects speed of processing and cognitive efficiency in general. There might be changes at the metabolic level, changes in the ways that neurotransmitters work to efficiently send along neural impulses.
>
> This injury doesn't show on structural tests, yet I infer that it is primary and organic, as opposed to psychiatric, emotional and behavioral. Emotional fallout is to be expected, but is likely secondary to the event (motor vehicle accident) that precipitated the significant change in brain function/life circumstance.
>
> That is the framework out of which I practice, although there are others – whom I respect – who think differently. Evidently [Dr. X's] view is different, or has evolved to reflect a more distinct distance from my framework.

So, after 24 months, the trust I had in Dr. X was shattered.

Problems with diagnosis

The injured brain as outdated computer

An unfortunate dynamic was at work during my various meetings with members of my recovery team that I believe contributed to Dr. X's misdiagnosis. My struggles to recover from most of my appointments were epic. Recovering from the Neuropsychological Evaluation is especially vivid, even though I had taken it spread out over three partial days. I suffered headaches and nausea and needed to lie down for several days afterwards.

Lynne wrote:

> I accompanied my husband on this visit with [Dr. X] because of my concerns about his depression, and because John tries to be upbeat and optimistic he often does not communicate just how bad he feels so much of the time.

Lynne and I tried to explain to Dr. X that the tests themselves, and my upbeat determination to do well on them, might have created a perception problem. It made me think that a survivor's brain can be compared to an outdated computer:

- The doctor sees the patient processing information, but might not see or fully appreciate the extreme effort of answering questions.

- The doctor also does not see the patient immediately after leaving his office and the "over-heating" that occurs for the rest of the day.

- It is not lost on the patient that the marketplace has no place for outdated computers that overheat after using. The patient is no longer "industry standard."

The outdated computer metaphor works to some extent: I present myself as upbeat and positive, and can answer basic questions. My brain appears to be functioning well. However, as a result of the effort the interaction requires, when I leave the doctor's office my outdated computer – my injured brain – "crashes."

I would return home from a visit to Spaulding with my brain "circuits" seriously overheated. I felt depleted, and recovering from these efforts

generally took several days. In hindsight, I regret that my recovery team –
particularly Dr. X – did not know the extent of my crashes following our
meetings.

A red, yellow and green stoplight

One consequence of presenting well is how an insurance company interprets a
doctor's notes. If the doctor uses generic terms such as "exhausted" without
specifying the extreme and unique cognitive exhaustion a TBI causes, an
insurer can conclude that certain tasks, or day-to-day living, are manageable
rather than debilitating.

With regard to a survivor's ability to return to work, think of it this way:

- <u>Red light</u>: The TBI patient reports a range of sequelae to the Attending
  Physician.

- <u>Yellow light</u>: The doctor uses bland, non-TBI specific language to record
  the sequelae, such as "fatigued," "tired," "trouble concentrating,"
  "irritable," "memory lapses," "slight stuttering," and even, in the case of the
  eternally optimistic, "generally upbeat." To add insult to the injury, it is
  common for doctors to preface sequelae with "patient complains of . . ."
  which sounds as though the patient's "complaints" do not represent an
  objective truth, but rather a statement subject to scrutiny and skepticism.

- <u>Green light</u>: An insurer's decision to force a TBI patient back to work by
  denying long-term disability benefits has huge implications, not only
  financially but for the prospects of the survivor's recovery.

Doctors should know that appearances can be deceiving

After one appointment with Dr. X, I went to the hospital cafeteria to have
lunch before my next appointment. I checked e-mail on my laptop, skimmed

the *New York Times*, and from all appearances, looked perfectly normal. Dr. X walked in and we waved, both of us smiling.

After another appointment with him, I was again waiting in the cafeteria when he walked in with a staff psychiatrist. I smiled and waved to both of them; they waved back. During my next appointment with Dr. X he asked me if a psychiatrist could sit in on our meeting, and I consented. When he wrote in his final report that my sequelae were attributable to sleep apnea and depression – not to a TBI – I wondered if the normal image I presented in the cafeteria had given them something to talk about.

So be aware that appearances can be deceiving. This might sound ridiculous, but if you have mild TBI and "look great," you might consider leaving the building between your appointments. You don't want to give any members of your recovery team a false impression. Most medical professionals have a harsh workload and, let's face it, human nature being what it is, appearances count for a lot. One day, with a lot more education about the condition, survivors of mild TBI will be able to come out from the shadows of a self-imposed exile, but until then, sometimes looking great works against us.

9 – Work Case Study: Heather

HEATHER WALKS HER DOG

"I felt like a duck, calm on the surface, feet paddling constantly underwater."

TBI survivors face the "you look great!" problem all the time. Heather e-mailed me enthusiastically after watching "You Look Great!" on YouTube. She had been a graphic designer for a commercial real estate company before her accident. Her experience with mild TBI is worth considering in some detail because it illustrates the workplace obstacles that survivors can expect to encounter.

Heather developed detailed books and maps that conveyed demographic information. On weekends, she trained for Half Iron Man events. On Easter Sunday of 2009 she took Moe, her sister's dog, out for a run in Albany, New York to train for an event in Rhode Island. Two minutes out from her sister's house, she fell on her face:

> I was running down the side of the road facing traffic and a car was coming towards me and I didn't know what Moe would do, so I put both my hands on his leash to hold it tighter and with both my hands down towards my waist I tripped and fell on my left eyebrow. That's what did it. I lay there for a second and I heard the car stop and the driver checked on me and told me I was bleeding. He made sure I got back to my sister's house.

> My self-awareness at that point, I didn't have a lot of it, but I did know that Natasha Richardson had recently died because she hit her head and didn't go to the hospital. So I went to ER. They ran me through a

> CT scan to check for fractures around my eye and I got stitches and
> was kind of loopy.

The next day Heather returned to work. At first her co-workers were sympathetic because she had a dramatic black eye and three stitches in her eyebrow. "People saw that and let me be." Meanwhile, as the outward signs of her injury began to heal, Heather began to show the symptoms of an injured brain:

> There were a couple different things. I was getting lost driving to
> work. And then I got lost in a stairwell at work. I kept my sense of
> humor about this. I'd come into the office and tell a co-worker and
> she'd say, "That's not right."
>
> Another thing was, there was a project I'd been working on that week,
> and somebody asked me, "What's going on with this project?" And I
> had absolutely no clue. It was like, I have no idea what you're talking
> about!

After the obvious signs of her injury healed completely, she found herself "in a bit of a pickle" because although she looked better, she felt worse. Her performance deteriorated.

Heather in a pickle

Many of Heather's work tasks required sequencing, and she was finding that kind of thinking increasingly difficult to do. Before her injury, if she was launching a big project she would say to herself, okay, I have to do this, this, and that, and I have to check in with so-and-so at points here, here and there. After the injury she struggled to figure out what step one was, and then she would have to ask herself, what's the next step? Instead of easily identifying the first ten steps, she struggled through each one.

She also discovered that her internal clock was "knocked off," making it almost impossible for her to determine whether a particular step was taking her two minutes or two hours. In a workplace environment driven by tight deadlines, this was a serious handicap.

She was also suddenly very "binary," seeing the world in either black or white – "there was no shade of gray" – and felt either very happy or very sad. She cried easily for no apparent reason, shocking her colleagues.

Communication breakdowns

Heather e-mailed co-workers repeatedly to explain how the injury was affecting her ability to work, and included Wikipedia articles on TBI and other resources to help them understand the challenges she was facing. "But they would just kind of…come at me with the same sort of big requests I had before the accident."

She persisted in her efforts to try to explain her condition to them and to her superiors, but they just didn't get it. To a large extent this was because she looked normal. "There's no doubt about that," Heather says. Her normal appearance was "most definitely" an obstacle to their understanding because mild TBI had not put her in a wheelchair or a brace or consigned her to crutches or a walker or left her spastic. The total absence of any visual evidence of an injury left her boss perplexed, irritated and skeptical.

Presenting well but grinding down

Before she worked for the real estate company, Heather had served with the Air Force's Elite Guard, working to protect nuclear missiles in Wyoming and Air Force generals on bases across Europe. This background actually compounded her problems. Her intense training for this high-level work had taught her how "to project a stable demeanor" in extreme situations, but this was precisely what might have deepened any doubts her boss and colleagues might have harbored about her injury.

She believes that her training actually hurt her because she should have "crawled into a corner" to recover. "I felt like a duck, calm on the surface, feet paddling constantly underwater."

Doing as little as possible goes against her grain

The injury afflicted her to the point where she "didn't even feel safe crossing the street" and was "overcautious," a fairly common behavior for people with TBI. She also grew concerned about her judgment:

> I have two dogs and one of them is fifteen and she's not quick and I was worried that if I tried to cross the street, I'd not have seen something to the left. A friend and I were walking down the street and he's aware of my injury and he told me I tried to walk into an intersection twice. It's like I wasn't fully aware of things that could cause me damage.

Her job and her anxieties about the quality of her work began to grind her down. "I remember a day when I think I came back [home] around 4; I told my boyfriend I was tired, and just went to bed." Heather's neurologist told her that struggling to perform the tasks associated with her job requirements "was not an ideal way to recover."

He urged her to do as little as possible and wrote a letter to her company boss explaining that her brain injury had left her with "severe emotional and cognitive problems":

> When I finally got my disability note I passed copies to my supervisor and other people who needed to have that information and when I gave it to the first person, she said, "This doesn't mean anything; what does this mean?"
>
> People didn't know how to handle me. I got shorter days. I had never been on disability, so I had no idea what I could or couldn't do in terms of just leaving. In the current economic environment, I was worried about losing my job.

Looking great confuses people

Like Heather, I have often wondered if my life would have been easier had the injury left a sign that immediately telegraphed my injury. Had I limped into my Case Manager's office and presented a droopy eye, spasticity and dramatically slurred speech, the insurance representative would have had no reason to doubt the reality of my TBI.

A man in his 60s with whom I work on our church council was in a terrible car accident 17 years ago. He walks and talks with extreme difficulty, but his mind is as sharp as it ever was when he worked as an engineer. It took a long time for me to understand his speech, and it is painful to even watch him walk with his double-crutches. He has taken great interest in my recovery because we are opposites in one important way. He confided in me, "John, I feel sorry for you." This really took me aback. He feels sorry for *me*? He explained that his injury is so obvious that people don't expect him to be as smart as he is. My injury, though, led people to expect the world from me, and he knows I can't deliver.

As Heather says:

> I think I am just going to start wearing a helmet in public. When my black eye went away and my stitches were gone there was nothing to show I had real problems. A helmet would make my invisible injury visible.

The invisibility of the injury confused her family members and friends as well, who made "jokey comments" about Heather "being on vacation."

"They made remarks such as, 'Oh, I wish I could stay home all day and take naps.'" She tries not to let it bother her, but she has told them, "This is not vacation time." Heather's brother was skeptical about her injury. "My brother said to me, 'Your employer can't keep you forever,' and I said, 'Well, I can't even drive!'"

Heather's boss finally gave her a leave after he spoke with Heather's neurologist, who helped him understand the severity of Heather's problem. Though she feels "quite guilty" about missing work, she also expresses a lot of anxiety about returning:

> I gave [my employers] an update, but I don't talk to them a lot because it causes great stress, and in one instance I was crying on my boss's voice mail. They have recently sent a very formally toned letter talking about how "the Company" is concerned and wants to know my current status…I think I need more time, but am scared to voice that for fear that people will see that as me wanting to have vacation time.

Heather says that she is "trying to recover and be my best, but I fear that I am doing that for the wrong people." I asked her, "Who are the right people?" She said, "I was trying to get better so people at work could have me around. The right people for me to recover for are me and my family."

No happy ending for Heather

One day a letter from the office arrived asking her when she expected to return. Heather "freaked out" and "stressed out" about it. She had been to her neurologist several times but had absolutely no idea when she would be cleared to return to work. She was recovering at an imperceptible "snail's pace," if at all. She didn't know how to begin to respond to the letter, so she did nothing:

> I couldn't pick up the phone. I couldn't write back. I couldn't think of another alternative. Just thinking about it reduced me to tears. It should have been no surprise when I received a letter later that said my position within the company was terminated because of "abandonment." This also took away my work disability payment. No job. No paycheck. I was numb.

One of Heather's friends recommended that she contact a lawyer, but it was too late. The lawyer informed her that, "because you didn't keep up communication, they have the right to terminate." She asked me, "What do I do now?" And I had no idea what to say to her.

10 – Work: From MVP to Nobody

ON THE OUTSIDE LOOKING IN

Four years into my injury, as I walked through the streets of New York's Upper West Side in the night rain, I stood facing a storefront window. In front of me was one of Fidelity's Investment Centers, closed, but well lit and immaculate. For many years Fidelity had entrusted me with a badge that I would use to swipe my way into some rather highly secured offices. True, I had earned that trust, but here I was now, brain-injured, on the outside looking in, knowing that that part of my life was most likely over.

The feeling of loss and loneliness reminded me of the time I was about to meet my friend and former colleague for lunch in Boston. I got to the intersection near the office a little early and realized how hard it would be to run into anyone I knew from the office. I dreaded the thought of stammering while trying to answer such hard questions as, "How are you?" I walked to a nearby storefront where I would have a good view of the intersection. I used to walk down the halls of the office happy and proud of my work and reputation, and here I was slinking around hoping not to see anybody I knew.

The dream

About a year after my injury I had a really vivid dream: I was attending some kind of big corporate training or marketing event in an elegant conference center. As people milled around waiting to be seated, I noticed that they all dressed in suits or expensive business-casual attire. Everyone was smarter, taller and 20 years younger than me. I tried to act casually to fit in, but I was shirtless and wore shorts. I didn't know anybody and nobody spoke to me, and I walked around feeling ashamed and embarrassed. I wanted to disappear.

I saw name tents placed on the tables in the main conference room and watched as people began to seat themselves. I hoped my own seat was off in a corner somewhere, but not only was my name tent up front, I had no chair, and everyone else had really nice chairs. I began to hunt for one and was about to grab a nice one from another room, but then somebody handed me one of those cheap folding chairs made out of canvas. It was torn and dirty, but I took it.

At that point I couldn't bring myself to sit around a table with people who radiated so much confidence and class, so I wandered down a hallway. A pretty woman walked towards me and then past me, and when I realized she had said hello I turned around and said, "Oh, hi." But she kept walking and then I clearly heard someone say to her, "He has a brain injury."

What was that all about?

You don't have to be a professional to interpret my dream. Before the injury, I was at the top of my game as a senior-level Instructional Designer. After the injury, even 20 minutes of concentrating left me reeling. My dream percolated from my deepest uncertainties about the loss of my work and what other people thought about me. Many mild TBI survivors report similar feelings, feelings that easily lead to depression.

Now, if I mess something up even slightly, I have been known to say with some bitterness and humor, "How the mighty have fallen!"

WORKING HARD WITHOUT EMPLOYMENT

Similarly, before the traumatic brain injury that Mike (Chapter 2) sustained in his terrible fall, he was at the top of his game professionally. Mike now heard many mornings from his wife, "Are you better? Do you think maybe today you'll have a productive day at work?"

He isn't better, and chances are he isn't going to get better. Mike knows that his wife looks at him and wonders how he can be disabled when he looks so normal. It can be difficult, especially at first, for even a spouse to "see" TBI. We don't look as though we have anything wrong with us so why don't we just get up, get dressed and go back to work?

Late one Sunday evening after Lynne and I shared dinner with a group of friends, somebody finally said, "Well, I've got to get up and go to work tomorrow!" Everybody but me said, "Yeah, me too," or "I hear ya!" Although my recovery team warned me against it, I could feel frustration, shame and even despair well up inside of me. The truth is I was working harder every day than I ever worked before the injury to try to recover. I should have felt proud about that.

What I did, and what I can't do

To be clear and specific as I worked with my recovery team and my insurer, I prepared a list of my job requirements. The list illustrates all the areas that require robust creativity and logical analysis, and a lot of other skills in between, like thinking on my feet and getting a complete, fluent sentence out of my mouth. As I prepared the list, it hit me hard that I was probably not going back to work any time soon.

I then worked with my recovery team to make a list of the sequelae that impair my functioning. These excerpts will be familiar to anyone with a TBI, even a mild one:

- Extreme cognitive fatigue

- Concentration

- Trouble with organization and time management

- Speech (stammering, halting); difficulty putting ideas into words

- Memory

- Diminished problem-solving and decision-making

- Diminished multi-tasking ability (can focus only on one thing at a time)

I showed the complete list to one of my doctors in our first meeting, trying to be helpful and precise about my injury. He looked at me in exasperation and said, "There are 15 things here!" I was really surprised that he didn't even try to problem-solve with me. I looked back at him calmly and said, "Well, let's group them then, shall we?" In that moment I felt like the grown-up.

Missing the tangibles and intangibles of my lost profession

One time, a doctor spoke to me using a tone so condescending that I interrupted him. "Look," I said, "I know what it's like to be a highly valued player on a team." I explained passionately how much I missed my job and my colleagues – many of whom became close friends – and being valued professionally.

Understanding my life a little better before the injury, he began to speak with more respect and empathy. On the way home I figured out that I had reacted so strongly because I was still grieving the loss of a professional life that had given me dignity. My neurologist's failure to uphold my dignity hit a very raw nerve.

One day early on in my recovery I felt slightly less fatigued, and because I was reading a little again, I thought maybe I was finally getting well enough to be approved to return to work. Just then I overheard Lynne on the phone with a colleague discussing the same kind of project that I worked on "back in the day." Overhearing her side of the conversation drove home how incapable I was of interactions that required my active participation.

TBI survivors are often completely demoralized when they are not approved to return to work. Some say they miss the workplace simply because it structured their days and that, and without it, they flounder. My injury more or less structures my days, but many of us do long for the teamwork and camaraderie we enjoyed with our colleagues. We miss the happy clients, the congratulatory pats on the back from team members, and the thank you's from a respected manager or mentor, not to mention the financial stability, satisfaction and self-esteem that come with a paycheck.

"Islands in a big sea"

At some point I had to step down from a position I was really good at and that reminded me of some of my old skills. I was serving as president of our church's council, which meant leading monthly meetings. After I stepped down, my friend and pastor wrote this to an insurer to describe his observations of the toll in cognitive fatigue that I increasingly paid as a result of the neurotrauma:

> . . . the effort of concentrating before these occasions has been costing him more and more. He has to withdraw for days ahead, work in short spurts, and otherwise, rest. And the cost after these occasions has been steadily rising. He'll be virtually prostrate for days after. His speaking or his presiding are still truly excellent, but they are islands in a big sea and more and more isolated from each other as the months pass.

A judge's ruling: "Fully Favorable"

At my hearing, the Social Security judge stated that I would make an "unreliable" employee given what an average day is like for me. In all of my professional life I had never heard that word applied to me, and I certainly never would have thought of myself as unreliable in anything. But as I thought about it, I realized that "unreliable" is a good word for me now because I never know what I'm capable of on any given day.

THE "YOU LOOK GREAT" PROBLEM

Meeting with a long-term disability insurance field rep

Knowing that my demeanor and positive outlook on life can contrast sharply with people who present their brain damage in excruciatingly obvious ways, I was a little concerned about an upcoming meeting with the insurance field representative. The company was reviewing my application for continued long-term disability benefits, and she simply wanted to meet me and ask how my recovery was going.

I arranged to meet her in the presence of both Lynne and Beth Adams, my Case Manager. I believed that both of them would be able to ground my interview in reality as they knew it. For example, if I said I occasionally enjoy dinner with friends, Lynne would be sure to explain the severe toll that socializing takes on me. If I said that my brain simply shuts down after exerting itself, Beth could explain that this is typical for someone recovering from a TBI.

I really had no reason to be concerned about my normal appearance, although I do recommend having one or more caregivers join you for such an important interaction. Once I began answering a few of the representative's open-ended questions – requiring more than a simple yes or no – I inevitably demonstrated ample evidence of my injury. It wasn't pretty; let's just say I failed to answer the questions the way I would have before the injury. The representative was polite and observant, and it didn't take her long to "get it"; my cognitive capabilities had clearly taken a sharp fall as a result of my injury.

Revisiting Mike

Mike wrote a harrowing e-mail to me:

> Work is killing me even though I am down to two days a week. I wish
> I had broken my back instead, at least people wouldn't expect me to
> get up and walk each morning. I can't imagine five years from now. I
> mean this injury has cost me my friends, my health, my hobbies, and
> it's destroying my marriage.

Gregg avoids driving through town

Gregg had an experience similar to Heather's (Chapter 9). It was not obvious
to fellow firefighters that Gregg was as injured as he said he was. "Most people
that talk to me wouldn't know I have an injury unless they knew me early on,
before it occurred," he says.

During the first few months of the injury other firefighters told him how great
he looked but also made jokes that suggested Gregg was maybe exaggerating
his injury. A friend's wife said, "I could use some time off myself." Gregg
finally decided to:

> . . . avoid driving through the town where I worked because I didn't
> want [former co-workers] to see me and think, oh, he's driving around;
> why isn't he working? I worried that they might think I was cheating
> the system.

WHAT OTHER PEOPLE THINK

Is it really possible to be indifferent about what people think of you?

Picture this: You've been out of the office for about a year and you've been invited to dinner with a group of former colleagues. You're feeling guilty because your absence from the office has meant that some of these people have had to work a lot harder. Nevertheless, it's sheer pleasure to see them again. You're sampling some great wines – this is before you learn that alcohol for the brain-injured is a neurotoxin – and you make a huge effort to be your old funny self. When you leave at the end of the evening you leave happy, having had a lot of fun.

You know, however, that over the next few days you will pay for your cognitive exertions, pleasurable though they were. The next day your mind wanders, and you start thinking that one of your co-workers also reports to your manager, who is likely to ask, "How did John seem on Saturday night?" You find yourself wrestling with the thing that has preoccupied you for months: What do other people think?

One of my greatest challenges has been surmounting my anxieties about what other people think because I look normal and can behave for short periods as if I am normal. As we laughed together, my colleagues might well have thought, "What brain injury?" Yet for five days after that party I suffered a massive cognitive hangover. The first day I crashed on the couch all day, and in fact I must have looked comical with my C-pap (a sleeping device), earplugs and noise-canceling headphones on, my red sweatshirt pulled over my face.

It distressed me to think that anyone would wonder why I was not back at work. My longing to remain connected to my colleagues compelled me to try to see them socially. I arranged to have lunch with Christine, for example, at a Thai restaurant. She told me about her family and what was happening at work, and I brought her up to date on me. Just spending time with her allowed me to imagine that I could soon return to work, especially if we were teamed together again. I told my SLP Rick that even though an hour of work at Fidelity would set me back for days, I could at least say I was back at work.

"Performances"

I fixated on what other people thought about my "performances" at parties or other social occasions, such as a fundraising banquet I MC'd. One person came up to me after the banquet and said, "I wish I could write and deliver something like that." After the success of my MC speech, how could I tell him, or anyone, that I was unable to work? The truth was that serving as MC made me feel smart and competent, which I rarely feel day-to-day. But nobody saw me during the weeks of preparation when it felt like I was writing with a big chunk of my brain missing (write – crash – recover – write – crash – recover) or during the agonizing aftermath (complete cognitive crash).

It took a long time for me to figure out that my social compulsions, anxieties and defensiveness were almost entirely about the loss of self-esteem. In one of my many sessions with my Social Worker, I explained that I never thought I had attached my identity to my work. I've always been more about my family and friends. But – and this is huge – a big part of my identity has always been *that* I worked.

Whether out of bitterness or envy, two ugly features of the human condition, people make assumptions and sometimes-snide comments about jobless individuals. Then one day I was the guy who didn't have a job. This fact was one of the many motivators for my writing this book.

"What a waste"

One night as I lay in bed unable to sleep, I thought of the philosopher Isaiah Berlin lying in bed waiting to die. A friend asked if he was afraid of death. He said he was not afraid, "but what a waste." I was mulling over all the things I wanted to do, and felt I needed to do, and how I had to spend so much time lying down with a towel over my face and my ear plugs in for hours every day doing absolutely nothing. "What a waste," I thought.

When I told Lynne about this, she had a different spin on it. She said, "Maybe all those years you were using your talents and energies as an instructional designer were a waste." Well, that was certainly something to think about, as long as I was just lying there! What all those years were, I think, were preparation for what I'm doing now: recovering from a brain injury and communicating successes, challenges and outright failures to other survivors.

When I said this to an old friend, that some good was coming out of this injury, he asked, "Knowing what you know now, would you choose to have the injury?" I did not hesitate: "No, I would definitely not choose to have the injury." So maybe it's a good thing that some of these decisions are out of our hands.

Barbara Webster

"Many of us were at the top of our game or 'rising stars.' We feel we are just a piece of who we used to be."

Barbara Webster facilitates my brain injury support group. In 1991, a car skidded into hers on a snowy road, totaling her car. Fortunately she had her seatbelt on. Barbara says, "I looked okay – not a scratch on me. The hospital sent me home with Advil." It turned out she had a severe case of Temporomandibular joint disorder (TMJ) – neck, jaw and shoulder soft tissue injury – and "I thought I couldn't think because of the fatigue and pain." Her brain injury remained undiagnosed for two years.

Twenty years later, she reports that she has made "great strides, but feel like I function at about 50 percent potential much of the time [and] continue to have significant difficulties with fatigue, speed of processing and sensory hypersensitivities." She found her inability to work to be especially harrowing.

> My major health problems have functioned as turn signals for my life, causing me to reevaluate my priorities and purpose, guiding me toward the ways I could best use my gift.

The root for the word "vocation" is *vocare*, which is the Latin for "to call – a summons from God to an individual or group to undertake the obligations and perform the duties of a particular task or function in life: a divine call to a place of service to others…that involves the total orientation of one's life and work in terms of one's ultimate sense of mission."[9] As Barbara observed, TBI survivors "need a whole new set of values and skills now, to make sense of our lives."

Barbara perfectly expresses what many of us feel:

> My identity used to be strongly attached to my accomplishments.
>
> If I couldn't do what I used to be able to do – who was I? We are embarrassed that we can't be and do and function as we used to.
>
> We have lost a lot of who we were.
>
> Many of us were at the top of our game or "rising stars." We feel we are just a piece of who we used to be.
>
> My self esteem was gone, I felt my life had no value because I couldn't work like I used to.

Barbara said that she had to do some serious soul searching to come to believe her life had value even if she couldn't do what she used to do: "I had to decide what was most important to do with my life, given my limitations. I had to find new ways to feel useful, or learn to value more other ways to feel useful. This took some time." It took me time too, but it's becoming clearer with every survivor I meet, and every new bond I make.

FACING THE PROSPECT OF NOT RECOVERING

"What strength do I have, that I should still hope? What prospects, that I should be patient? Do I have the strength of stone? Is my flesh bronze? Do I have the power to help myself, now that success has been driven from me?" Job 6:11-13

The odds of recovery are vastly in our favor

Four months into the injury, I asked the neurosurgeon, "What if I don't get better?" and "What if I improve but then plateau short of full recovery?" He put my chances at full recovery within a year at 90%, but said that there tends to be diminishing returns; the longer it takes to heal, the less healing will occur.

The longer it takes for survivors to see improvements, the fewer improvements they will see.

(Note: When I mentioned this to Rick Sanders, he said that Spaulding is revising their view of the window of recovery to two to three years, or even more.)

The neurosurgeon added that the longer it takes, the less likely that I'll fully recover. Then he said: "Frankly I'm discouraged at your progress. Many people would have fully recovered by now."

But then, surgeons are not noted for their bedside manners.

A shock at what I'd lost

Almost a year into my injury, Lynne had me try something from one of her projects to test my reading comprehension. All I had to do was read six short training modules and answer six multiple-choice questions at the end of each one. I read through the first module fairly well and should have breezed through the questions. I missed one of the general understanding questions. I began reading the second module and stared at the first screen for five minutes.

I had not burst into tears since beginning 20 mg of the antidepressant Celexa about 8 months after my injury, but it really disturbed me that I could not make sense of the content on the first screen. I told Lynne about it, and said I felt no different than if I had attempted this six months before. Not only was I stalled, like a lawn-mower on long grass, but I felt physically ill, actually nauseous. I wanted to persist, thinking if I gave it more time the content would sink in, but I got worse. Lynne wisely closed the laptop.

How I came to think about resuming my career

In the first year, the prognosis for my recovery seemed good because the MRI, CT scan and EEG were all clean, even though I knew that the brain's damage does not always show up on these tests. I asked Beth Adams how the decision was going to be made about my return to work because I felt anxious about it, and frankly it was awkward talking to people who saw me on a good day because I thought they might be thinking, "Now why can't you work?" She said, "Don't put that on yourself in addition to everything you're going through. Say that your recovery team has not okay'd you to go back to work." That has helped.

Here's how I pictured my chances of returning to my profession:

Figure 3:

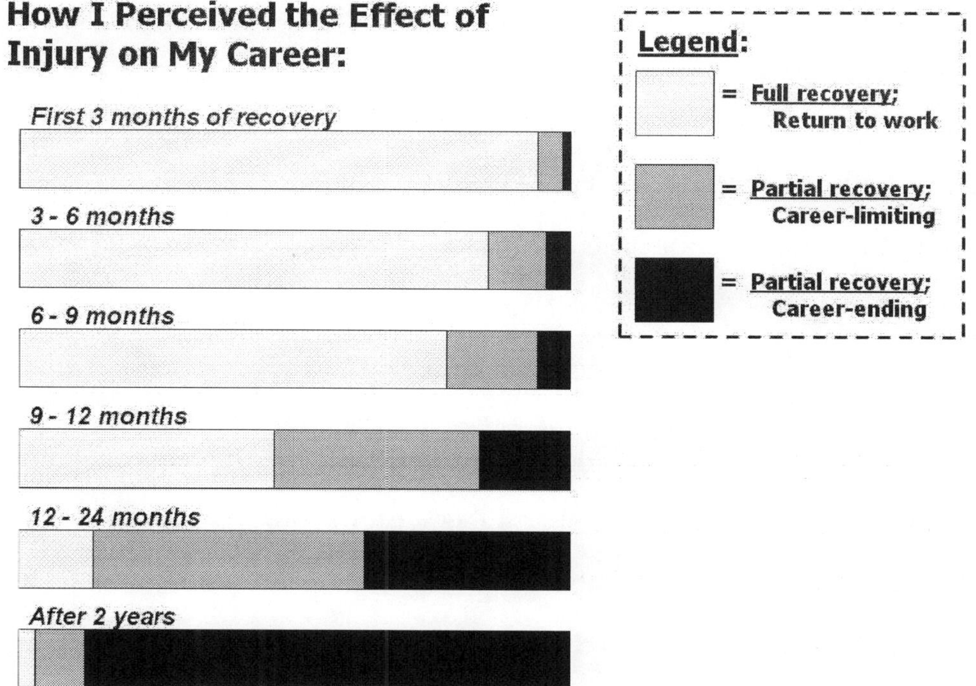

As the months passed, especially after the first year, it simply became less likely that my brain was going to heal back to normal – normal for me, anyway. The chart is not scientific; it is just my perception.

It's important to note that when I told Lynne I didn't think I'd ever have a career again, she disagreed. She said I would just have a different career. These are words to live by. And maybe that is the difference between recovery and rehab. Recovery means returning to work and your old life. Rehab is adjusting to a new life.

YOUR JOB AND YOUR WORK

Your job is to get better

First of all, your job is to get better; if you can't get better, your job becomes not to get worse. Your job is to learn and use strategies for living inside your brain injury in what is often an unintentionally hostile environment, the world of noise, stimulation, complexity and stress.

Your work is to reach out

If your *job* is to get better, your *work* is to help someone who has not had the injury as long as you and is without your experience, resources and strategies. Reach out and make that person's recovery better than yours has been. That person needs you, and – think about this hard – you need that person.

Peter, a friend of mine, asked to have breakfast with me after hearing my presentation at a church group, one that emphasized the theme of God and suffering. A devout Christian, he had spent years as a doctor among radical Muslims in Indonesia. In a time of escalated tensions and violence directed at

Christians, he escaped with his head on his shoulders when others were less fortunate. He literally jumped on a boat chased by a mob wielding machetes.

His new line of work is at an emergency room working the night shift. His stories are gut-churning to us milder types. With typical honesty and no false modesty, he says he likes the job a lot and he's good at it. As we talked about my injury and painfully slow recovery, he spoke to me not only as a friend but as a brother in the Christian faith. Familiar with pain and suffering, he was gentle with me and – even though I looked great – heard my speech and knew that I was faltering.

When I shared the awkwardness of not returning to my job while all my friends are hard on work every day, Peter – bless his heart – said I had much to teach my friends about "work" and its role in our lives, and that some people work to excess to avoid doing what God really wants them to be doing.

Looking back now I remember that for at least a year before my injury I prayed very specifically about the work of my life. I prayed, in essence, "God, I'm happy doing what I'm doing. I work with great people, the work is very creative and challenging, it pays well and I am proud of my reputation. But is this what you want me to be doing? I am in your hands." As they say, be careful what you pray because the answer might be hugely different from anything you could have imagined.

Vocation, and what it means to be human

An essay on vocation and what it means to be human is beyond me at this point in my recovery, but I will list some thoughts to consider. You might want to talk about them with your caregiver, or bring them to your brain-injury support meeting and engage other survivors in this conversation.

We are what we eat, but we are not what we work

For the sake of our sanity and our recovery, and to re-affirm our lives, we must recognize our value apart from the things we do, apart from accomplishments. Our worth is not based on what we *do* but on who we *are*. Mere achievement – our performance – is not what makes us valuable human beings. We must believe this if we lose the ability to achieve and perform.

I had lunch recently with a former colleague whose whole sense of worth, it seemed to me, was wrapped up in the company he had started 20 years ago. He was spending himself for the sake of that company, and measured the success of his life by the success of the company.

As I drove home, I thought, "I wonder how he would do with a brain injury. How would he think of himself if he couldn't accomplish what he was used to accomplishing on any given day of his professional life?" We must be convinced of our worth beyond our accomplishments.

What is your piano?

Unless the biopic starring Jamie Foxx horribly misled us, Ray Charles was blind, yet played the piano brilliantly. What is *your* piano? Beethoven[10] was deaf and yet wrote symphonies. What is *your* symphony? I decided a year after my injury that this book would be my symphony. Do you need an intermission?

Tom Today

Tom (Chapter 2) is currently employed by a small agency that serves the mentally ill and he finds the work deeply satisfying. Massachusetts state vocational rehabilitation counselors steered him to the work after extensive testing. He says:

> I'm happy because of where I am today. The disability has changed my life completely, but I've learned to become an advocate for the mentally ill. I teach people how to get back to work. So there's a reason for everything.

He adds that when everybody in the agency goes to lunch, despite the fact that "these are my own people," he is unable to sit in the cafeteria because he still can't cope with crowds. He is content. "I have a rewarding and fulfilling job that makes me cry tears of joy."

11 – Work-Related Strategies

INFORMAL ADVICE

Having learned of her reputation in the field, I contacted a prominent medical center professor and director, who recommended the following strategies regarding returning to work:

> You might choose to work with a neuro-trauma rehabilitation professional or a neuropsychologist to manage your recovery and return to work.
>
> An approach that we have found to be most helpful in assisting patients with recovery and with return to work is as follows:
>
> 1. Injured person obtains a note from the **attending physician**, confirming that an injury has occurred, and which states patient has not yet been medically cleared to return to work. Hopefully patient can use sick leave to cover this time.
>
> 2. Patient **follows all recommended medical advice and treatment** during these early days of recovery, e.g., medications for headache if appropriate, pacing of activities, rest, light exercise, to see how symptoms resolve. There should be significant improvement within the first few weeks, with further significant improvement during the next 60 days.
>
> 3. During this time of early recovery, the person can also consult with a **vocational counselor familiar with mild TBI**, who can assist with contacting person's HR Dept, etc., if the person is going to need a gradual return to work, some accommodation while continuing to recover, etc. Even if it is not yet known what the patient might need, the vocational counselor can help get the needed info, and reduce stress on the patient.

4. If this is a more complicated mild TBI the patient should ask their attending MD for a referral to some **outpatient neuro-rehab care**. It is likely to take this person longer to recovery.

As part of the **neuro-rehab referral** for such things as Speech (cognitive rehab), PT (balance, pain), Rehab Psych (for support while coping and vocational help), a neuropsychological evaluation (NPE) would be indicated at +three months post injury if the injured person is not doing well. The NPE results can help guide the cognitive and psychological care as well as vocational planning. The physician will guide the PT if needed.

The vocational counselor is the person who can help work out a short-term **medical leave** if needed, with the support and agreement of the MD.

Arthur has two pieces of advice

When it comes to employers after an injury, Tom's partner Arthur (Chapter 2) advises two things:

1. Don't assume your employer will cover you

Avoid making assumptions about your employer's disability plans, your coverage, and their perception of the injured partner. Even though Tom's former employer is a 152 billion dollar corporation we had to fight for every payment and ultimately Tom's disability coverage from the company's insurer was cancelled. The insurance person was the one who said to Tom, "It's not like you got your eye poked out."

2. Work with your state rep to get vocational rehabilitation

> Massachusetts Senator John Kerry failed to respond to any of our letters. It wasn't until we contacted our state rep that we got some real help. She got Tom's vocational rehab going.

Heather's (Chapter 9) work-related strategies

Strategy	Explanation
Do NOT return to work until your Attending Physician says you are ready.	I should not have tried to return to work with an injured brain and neither should you. You recover by resting your brain. You do NOT recover by fretting over unfinished projects at work or by stressing out about insurance paperwork. I should have involved my doctor (and other professionals) in all my decision-making about work right from the start.
If you do return to work, watch for signs that you may be pushing your brain too far	When I first went to my neurologist, I had to have help filling out my own health forms, and that should have signaled me that I was not ready to return to work. I just didn't see it. At work I couldn't keep track of anything I was supposed to be doing, so I tried using sticky notes and had a whole desk full of them. I couldn't keep track of time and had problems with sequencing, so I'd forget to look at the previous piles of sticky notes. The accumulating "To Do's" overwhelmed me. In addition I was perpetually looking for my car keys, got lost on the way to work, and couldn't make my meetings with colleagues on time. The problem with trying to recover while you work is that you might see certain signs that you are getting better, but you can't tell if you are getting back to normal. And there's a big difference between getting better and getting back to normal. I should have assumed that I needed to rest my brain.

Heather's work-related strategies, cont'd

Strategy	Explanation
Work with your doctor to keep your employer informed of your progress.	Consider allowing your boss or supervisor to initiate a call to your doctor about your situation. Just be sure to inform your doctor first. I should have discussed my work situation with my doctor right away and asked him to communicate directly with my employer about the effects of my brain injury.
Have your doctor write a letter to your supervisor.	The doctor's letter should make these points: 1) You are unable to work at this time due to a traumatic brain injury. 2) There is no timeline for recovery from this type of injury. 3) I will keep you informed about her progress. Call me if you have questions. So the point is not lost on your employer, you might also write a letter for their files that communicates similar points: Dear (boss), I am unable to work at this time due to a traumatic brain injury. My doctor has declared that I am disabled and has not cleared me yet to return to work. There is not an accurate timeline for recovery. I ask for your kindness/consideration during this stressful and worrisome time for me and my family.

Heather's work-related strategies, cont'd

Strategy	Explanation
Identify someone who can maintain regular communication with your employer and your doctor, and monitor communications between your employer and your doctor.	You must avoid company accusations of "abandonment," which will cost you disability insurance and other benefits. There is so much stress, anxiety and confusion in the aftermath of a brain injury that it's simply too difficult for a survivor to handle these things effectively. Communications, whether e-mail, snail mail or phone calls, with work supervisors can be as simple as: "Dr. A has not yet cleared Jane to work because of the disability caused by her traumatic brain injury. Dr. A will inform you when Jane is able to return to work. If you have questions, Dr. A can be reached at _____."
Document all communications.	Make duplicate copies of all e-mail and snail mail correspondence. Take notes on all phone calls, and include dates. File documentation in an orderly fashion. Documentation is critical to any legal steps that you may take down the road.
Remember that you are not lazy or stupid. You are injured.	Respect your injury by getting help when you need to.

12 – Loss of Self, and Depression

"The spirit of a man will sustain his infirmity; but a wounded spirit, who can bear?" Proverbs 18:14

LOSING WHO WE WERE

Like it's a lifejacket, I tug on tight to my conviction that I am still the same person I was before TBI. Another survivor I know firmly maintains that she is very much the same person she was before her accident, and resists any suggestion that her essential personality or essence has dramatically changed.

But different survivors feel as though they've landed at various places along the spectrum of being the same person and being a new person entirely. Elizabeth and Mike find themselves down on the pavement looking up dazed and reeling at the truck called TBI that hit them.

Elizabeth

Still longing to be the person she once was, Elizabeth describes the indelible day of her car crash a year before:

> I remember a car cutting me off at the intersection, and slamming my brakes on. And I remember suddenly seeing the car right on the tail of the car that my bumper had just missed and we were about to hit hard head-on. And I remember that moment, when sounds suddenly hush, and reality starts to drown out, time rather freezes, and you are bitterly alone with that voice in your head: "This is happening." And you surrender. You have no choice. Life as you know it is not in your hands.

So I clenched the wheel as tight as I could, as if I had super powers to brace myself and dissuade harm. I clenched my eyes as well, never knowing I would never open them as myself again.

That is how I died.

Mike

"How do you mourn the loss of yourself?"

Mike told me about one of the times he and his wife had argued about his inability to work. Knowing how difficult it is for a TBI survivor to sustain an argument with anybody, especially with a spouse, I asked him what happened.

Mike said in a fit of anger he went from room to room turning face down every photo of himself taken before the accident. As he told me what he had done, he sounded crippled with shame and grief. "How do your mourn the loss of yourself?" he asked me.

I have thought of his question many times, and the subject of loss of self comes up a lot with the brain injured. We are not who we were – that person is gone – and we miss that person intensely. We talk about our lives in terms of "before" and "after" the injury.

Mike wrote to me:

I have been crushed. Life's going 100 mph and I am in the slow lane with my hazards on.

John, I truly feel disabled…I don't know where you found the acceptance of this hand we've been dealt but I wish I had just half of it. I hate the loneliness. I was thinking the other day that it has been almost two years since I have looked anyone in the eye and how lonely you feel without eye contact. That's why I am getting a dog. They don't care what's wrong with you…Man's best friend.

As for the cure, a cure, any cure. I don't think it exists. An escape does exist if you find a way to shut off your brain, the way you do when you exercise or do some mindless routine. I think the escape is to fill the day with as many of these tasks that enable us not to think.

The more I read about TBI the more I think we are f---ed.

As a result of his crippling sequelae, Mike could no longer work. Sometimes he still goes into the office because he has nowhere else to go, although there is almost nothing that he is capable of doing there. Other times he'll sleep, but most of the time, he'll just sit there. We can only imagine what is going through his head.

Your life begins to unravel no matter who you think you are

No matter whether you think you are basically the same person as you were, or you think that person is no more, today's fact is that you probably feel lousy and you are having another terrible day. You can't do things you used to do, and the things you can do don't bring you pleasure anymore. You often feel sad and lonely, one day leads to the next, and all of that wears you down.

Besides these "intangibles," the chemistry in your brain might have been altered by your injury and the functioning compromised – say, communication between your pituitary and hypothalamus – and you might begin experiencing clinical depression. Learn how to watch for it, and take steps to deal with it before you begin believing that this new life is not worth living.

THE ONSET OF CLINICAL DEPRESSION

"I am fighting a fixed bout every day and keep fooling myself I'll go 12 rounds."
Mike

Before my injury I had never suffered from clinical depression. As I started to read about brain injury I learned that depression quite often followed, so I kept a sharp eye out for it. In the first year I was reluctant to admit that I was depressed. I was frustrated, yes. I was sad and lonely, yes. But as I entered my second year, knowing that my chances for full recovery were diminishing, I started paying closer attention to the signs.

According to the National Institute of Mental Health, signs of depression might include the following:

- Difficulty concentrating, remembering details and making decisions

- Fatigue and decreased energy

- Feelings of guilt, worthlessness and/or helplessness

- Feelings of hopelessness and/or pessimism

- Insomnia, early-morning wakefulness, or excessive sleeping

- Irritability, restlessness

- Loss of interest in activities or hobbies once pleasurable, including sex

- Overeating or appetite loss

- Persistent aches or pains, headaches, cramps, or digestive problems that do not ease even with treatment

- Persistent sad, anxious, or "empty" feelings

- Thoughts of suicide, suicide attempts

Because many of these things come close on the heels of a TBI, you need to watch for the intensity and frequency of them.

For example, there's a difference between sadness and depression, frustration and depression, feeling worthless and depression. As feelings of sadness, frustration, and worthlessness intensify, you might well become clinically depressed. You need to recognize and address it. Because you are in the thick of it, you may need your caregiver or a loved one to help you recognize the signs.

Watch for signs

Journal entry

To provide a glimpse of a particularly bad day, here is an excerpt from my journal:

> Abnormally long time prone on bench swing . . . had hood over face and towel . . . some sleeping but lots of thinking and not moving. Lynne came out to see how I was doing and gently asked if I was okay . . . I'm very conscious of a new phase of my recovery (if you can call it recovery) . . . not sure how to explain it. I feel like withdrawing + not communicating. Maybe a doctor's advice wd be to DO LESS . . . relinquish tasks . . . I need more time every day in some kind of isolation tank. What's the difference betw that + being dead? Bcz I can get up periodically.

Figure 4:

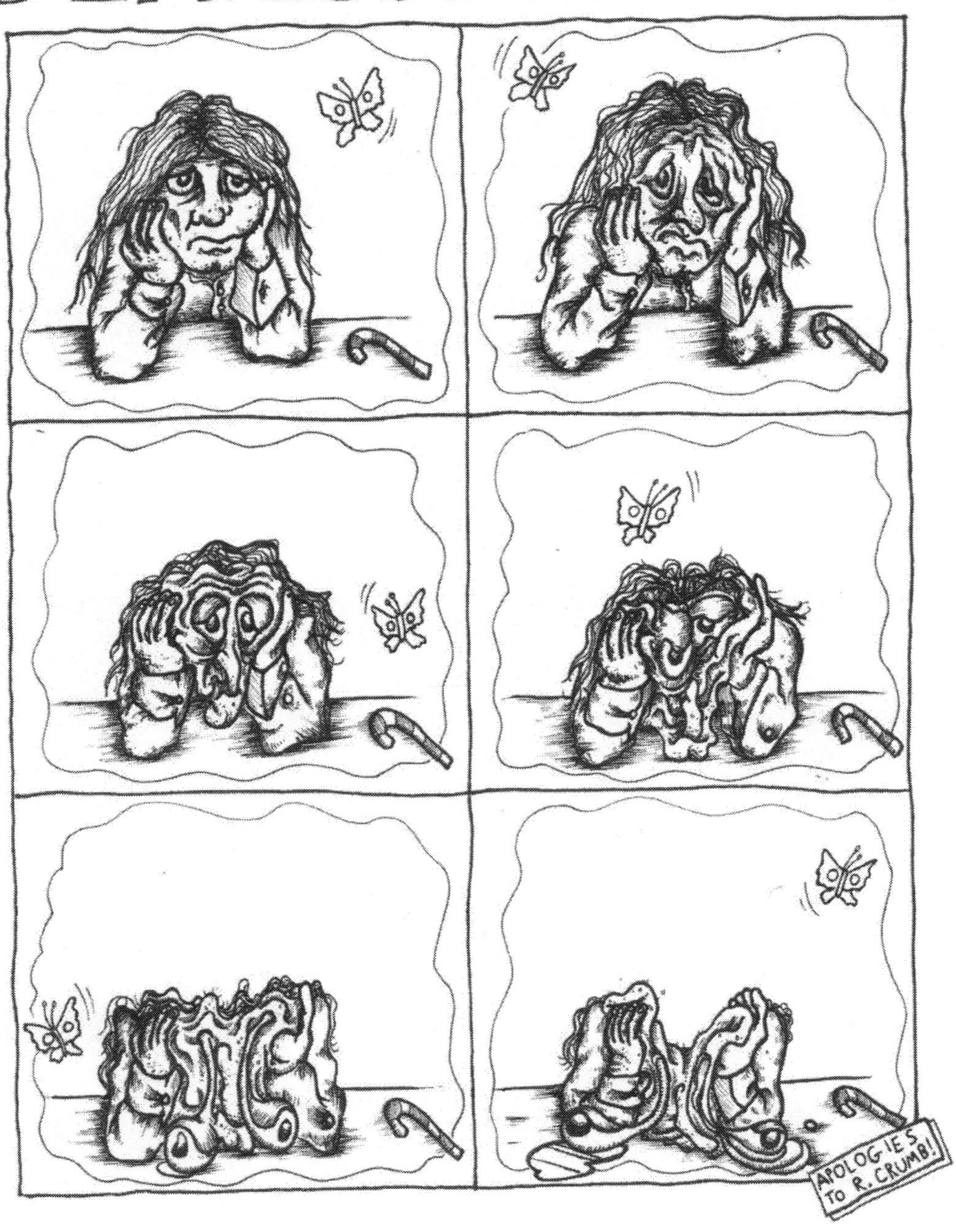

Artwork: Chris Byler

In a concerned letter to an insurer, Lynne wrote:

> When I see John with a towel over his face and plugs in his ears to shut out any mental stimulation at all – a man who before his injury was "in the superior range of intellectual functioning" – I can understand why he suffers bouts of depression just from the standpoint of frustration and despair over his condition.
>
> But more to the point, clinical depression is far more than the understandable frustration at being diminished.

During the months Lynne wrote about, I had become dependent on Concerta, a time-release stimulant, which kept me active when I should have rested and awake when I should have been sleeping:

> Over the past 18 months or so I have watched my husband's condition slowly deteriorate. My concerns have been growing as I have watched him try to pace his daily activities and continue to slog through the debilitating and demoralizing effects of the brain injury, even as these effects take a greater toll on him.
>
> For the first time since John's injury, I have seen behaviors and heard dark phrases that worry me greatly. Because TBI has taken from him so much of life's pleasures, I often wonder about his will to go on. I have lost a lot of my confidence that he has the ability to – and can be trusted to – make the kinds of decisions that take into account his own health and safety, and that of our family.

The coffin

One very cold November evening Lynne and I had a difficult conversation about Will's use of the Internet. It wasn't an argument at all, just the normal give and take of opinions that parents have to sort through to arrive at a solution.

This stressed my brain, and I went out onto the screen porch to gather wood for the stove. I stood out there without a coat for half an hour, just feeling so sad. I stared at the box that holds our wood supply, and as my thoughts began to unravel, I reflected that the box looked like a coffin and thought how peaceful it would be to lie in it.

Lynne wrote about this incident to an insurer:

> John's Primary Care Physician wrote that "he denies suicidal ideations," but John's remark about the coffin alarmed me. In 26 years of marriage, this normally upbeat and positive man has NEVER alluded to suicide or fantasizing about death. John sometimes enters such a dark place in his head that lately I am unsure if I can trust him to safeguard his life.

Dark vocabulary

Alarming words and phrases crept into my vocabulary. Lynne told me I often said that I felt "absolutely immobilized," "paralyzed," "comatose," "disabled," "resigned to suffering," and that "everything is an effort." At one point I admitted to her that I was feeling defeated and morose and nihilistic, and I'd say stuff like:

- "I feel broken and defeated."

- "I've forgotten what it feels like to feel good."

- "I'm not looking for euphoria. I just don't want to feel terrible all the time."

- "I'm as sick as I've ever felt."

- Particular days are "killers" and "groaners."

- "I just want to do nothing."

- "I'm frustrated at being so diminished."

- "It pains me to think anyone wonders why I'm not back at work."

Despairing of full recovery

Sometime in the early winter of 2008 I began to despair that I would not fully recover. I told Lynne that I was very worried that my "wellness window" was getting narrower in the mornings – I used to feel better in the mornings and then decline throughout the day – and that sometimes I felt "devastated for most of the day." My despair forced me to retreat and lie down for longer periods.

After I visited Lynne's father at the hospital when he broke his hip, I told her that "I looked around and saw people in hospital beds with oxygen tubes and that's all I wanted to do . . . lie down, close my eyes and BREATHE."

Social isolation

Lynne confided to her sister that she thought I was manifesting textbook signs of depression. She then wrote to an insurer about my increasing desire for social isolation:

> John increasingly isolates himself because of the effort to be with other people, including members of his own family. Lately he has been saying that he is "feeling the need to drop out of society" and that he "can't think of any place I want to go – movies or to friends – because of the effort and the aftermath of the effort."
>
> John used to be lively and engaging and fun at dinner parties, but now he says, "I'm a real downer."
>
> One illustration: Towards the end of February 2008 we went to a dinner at our pastor's home with maybe ten other guests, and 15

> minutes into it John retreated to a back room where he sat staring at the rug for about 45 minutes. He called for me, we talked, and we agreed he should just go home and I would follow him later.

She soon confronted me with her fears, and I acknowledged that I was extremely depressed. We agreed I would bring it to my doctor's attention right away.

Celexa helped me

I brought my darkness to my doctor, whose notes read:

> Mr. Byler returns today for follow-up. He is feeling miserable on a daily basis . . . in general, he feels that he is so easily overloaded mentally that he does not have much quality of life. He does not want to see friends as much as before because he feels they have a dishonest interaction when he does not acknowledge the brain injury. He also finds it exhausting to socialize. He does admit to feeling somewhat depressed.
>
> It seems to me that Mr. Byler is significantly more depressed than I have seen him for some time.

He gradually increased my dose of the anti-depressant Celexa from 20 mg a day – initially prescribed for lability (sudden crying) – to 30 mg, then 40 mg, then 50 mg. Somewhere along the way, I cut it back to 40 mg a day, and that has been my dosage ever since. It has not erased my depression but it's given me a better baseline.

Sometime later the doctor wrote that "excessive mental exhaustion with mental activity continues to be a major problem," and that I no longer seemed to be depressed. Lynne, however, amended the doctor's observation to an insurer:

> On this particular day John told [the doctor] that he did "not feel depressed," but clinical depression is so deep rooted in John's life now he has learned to put a brave face on it, and a smile or a humorous remark might be misconstrued as a lack of depression. Living with John as I do, I know better than anyone what he faces and battles every day.

Recently, I consulted with my doctor about reducing the dosage from 40 mg, and went several days on 30 mg. I ended up feeling so awful that the reduced dosage was all I could think of as the reason. It didn't take any convincing to go back to 40 mg, and that seems to be just right.

Thinking better of admitting myself to hospital

About a month later I was having one of the lowest days in my recovery. I talked with Rick Sanders about the possibility of checking in to Spaulding because I really felt at the end of my rope. His notes read:

> Patient arrives despondent & teary today as he describes persistent symptoms of cognitive fatigue and somatic discomfort of a debilitating degree. He states he is 'a raw nerve' as if he is sunburned and the sun is everywhere. He notes that any activity demands cognitive resources and he is depleted.

Rick reminded me that an inpatient stay at a hospital like Spaulding can be cognitively taxing in and of itself, noisy and over-stimulating if what you really need is rest. I thought better of the idea and just went home and tried to make the best of it.

Madelaine Sayko

Madelaine Sayko, a prominent brain-injury advocate and educator, is another of my new friends. As we spoke about her book in progress, she explained that it will not be a memoir or a how-to-live-with-brain-injury guidebook. It will be more of a theory of change and resilience. I can't wait to read it. As we began to get to know each other, I found that she was much more sanguine or at least philosophical about this whole issue of the loss of self. She said it beautifully:

> I often say I live in a house without mirrors now – the familiar things that reflected who I was are gone and so I have to just believe who I am. I don't mourn, I don't look back, I don't recover. I rebuild, I hope, I look ahead.

Sayko strategies

She also offers some especially salient advice on preventing, or at least talking oneself down from, feelings of despair and hopelessness. She offers the following strategies:

- Have someone you trust, believe in, and care about help reinforce your strengths and abilities and gifts. In despair, people forget that they have any good parts.

- Have this person provide you with some perspective. This is also a skill that someone can teach people with TBI or who are depressed. How do you fix things? Look at your situation as if it were a mission, a project, a car that isn't working. Find the metaphor that makes sense so you can disassemble the problem, prioritize it and start fixing it. Problems often just seem too big to face – and they especially seem that way to someone with TBI.

- Focus on someone who admires you. Step outside of yourself and know that someone needs you. Focus on the self-worth that comes from this realization, rather than anxiety or guilt at the possibility of letting them down.

- Sometimes it is helpful to volunteer or do something for anyone else who is visibly struggling. This can help refocus your thoughts. *(My caveat: See Chapter 20 – Support Groups and Volunteering: Yea or Nay?)*

- Avoid intoxicants; especially if you are feeling dark and are alone. Most folks with brain injury struggle with impulse control, and intoxicants make this worse.

- Be kind to yourself. Nurture yourself. If you need to, it's okay to take to your bed for a day, lie on the floor in a patch of sunshine, or just sit quietly.

Memento vivere

As if that were not enough to sustain me, Madelaine also introduced me to a wonderful phrase: Memento vivere. It means simply, "Remember to live."

CONFRONTING THE ISSUE OF SUICIDE

Thoughts of suicide ("suicidal ideation")

One survivor I know started making the same comment every time I talked to him:

> I'm telling you John, I felt so bad if I had a gun I would have shot myself. Not really, but you know what I mean.

After about the fourth time he said it, I brought it to his attention. He doesn't say it anymore, but I really don't know if he still thinks it.

My own downward spiral begins with simply imagining swinging contentedly at the end of a rope: no more responsibility to do what you can't do, no more misunderstandings, no more failure and disappointments; just letting go and letting gravity do its work. But I always walk it back. I know full well that I have so much and so many to live for, and that my life is full of loved ones and loved experiences.

If ever you or a loved one is in a crisis of possibly suicidal proportions, visit the National Suicide Prevention Lifeline online, or call 800.273.TALK. Here is the best strategy I can share if you begin fantasizing about suicide:

Don't do it. It's not even an option. Treating the decision as though it's a toggle switch, as I did with alcohol, I picture it on the "off" position permanently. Sometimes having no middle register, no gray area, makes these things easier. There is no debate. (I generally like to think that I won.)

I was a guest on Craig Sicilia's radio show out of Spokane, Washington – Brain Injury Radio: The Silent Epidemic – to talk about this subject. The co-host, a former Marine officer, recounted his moving story about being in such a dark place that one day he put a gun to his forehead. He almost pulled the trigger, but then he thought, "Wait a minute. I'm a Marine. If I'm going to do this, I'm going to do it right." He put the gun down, walked upstairs and changed into his formal dress blue uniform. When he picked up the gun again, he saw himself in the mirror and was appalled at who looked back at him and what his life had come to. In that "time out," that brief interval, he changed his mind, with thoughts of his daughter in his head instead of that bullet.

Meds and suicide

Both the Marine officer, Kevin A. Phillips, and Craig Sicilia had disastrous experiences with medications, which actually seemed to create suicidal thoughts. Doctors often call these "suicidal ideations" in their notes. In Craig's case, early in his injury he simply told his doctor that he felt sad all the time. The doctor put him on a particular med and it was only then that Craig began to think seriously of suicide. When the doctor heard this development, he doubled the dose. This did not have the desired effect of lowering his suicidal ideations. Craig landed in an institution, the first of four stints there thinking simply that he wanted to die.

Fast forward to the present day, and both Kevin and Craig are off of anti-depressants and neither are plagued with suicidal thoughts. Having said that, the source of your clinical depression might be chemical, in which case your doctor might be able to prescribe exactly the right medication that will correct this imbalance. You will have some hard choices ahead of you, and I would advise against ruling out medication or doctors' care ahead of time. Keep an open mind about combating your depression with whatever remedies are available, whether pharmaceutical or homeopathic in nature.

Consider, too, that medication might simply improve your energy, not your darkest moods. In some cases, people in their depression are in such bad shape that they can't even get off the couch to get the gun in the next room to shoot themselves. After medication, if their depression doesn't lift but their energy improves they might now act on their darkest thoughts. This is another reason to decide carefully what course of treatment you will pursue.

Some survivors say that marijuana is the only thing that makes them feel better. They say it eases their depression considerably, and eliminates any thoughts of suicide. When I searched "TBI and cannabis," no shortage of interesting-sounding articles popped up:

- "Endocannabinoids and Traumatic Brain Injury"

- "The Therapeutic Potential of the Cannabinoids in Neuroprotection"

- "Cannabinoids as Therapeutic Agents for Ablating Neuroinflammatory Disease"

With my limited cognitive capabilities, I'm not the one to dive in to this complicated topic, and not only because they contain words like "ablating." Clearly, research should continue on the effects of cannabis on the quality of the TBI survivor's life, both day-to-day and long term. If results bear out this "grass-roots" anecdotal evidence, perhaps state laws on medical marijuana should be mellowed; I mean, relaxed.

Madelaine weighs in

Madelaine Sayko believes that suicide comes from feeling both unempowered and overwhelmed, "as though the situation is a tsunami that will drown you inevitably. Suicide seems like the less painful way to go – short and sweet." Although frequently warning signs flare up, it is equally true that suicide is a common, albeit fleeting notion for many people. For those with brain injury, however, the lack of impulse control combined with the physically and emotionally exhausting conscious effort of doing what was once effortless can make even a small event the tipping point.

But, she continues, those contemplating suicide must realize:

- You are still capable and you can be helped.

- You have meaning, and you have value to contribute to the world.

- Feelings of inadequacy are not character issues or weakness. "Have grace with yourself."

- Suicide is permanent.

She suggests that if you are going through a rough patch it might be worthwhile to post these truths on all your mirrors. Finally, Madelaine notes that the most important thing we can do is to stop hiding from the topic of suicide, and the issues of making mistakes and feeling like a failure.

> We must stop pathologizing emotion, fear, and shame. This means offering more than applause when someone says in front of an audience, "I tried to kill myself." It means offering them a job, trusting them, asking their advice, doing something with them, spending time with them, helping them figure out how to pay their bills, organize their house. Yeah, depressed people are a drag. But dead people are a bigger drag.

Affirm life

In Chapter 24 – The Possible Role of Prayer in Recovery – I sound the refrain, "Desperate times call for desperate measures." Come up with whatever deterrent you can think of. You must stop yourself from taking any action that would harm yourself or anybody else. In my case, even before the injury, when life got tough and my mind began to wander, all I had to do was think of my three sons getting dressed up in tie and jacket, Lynne wearing black and attending my funeral.

Let me state what to survivors is an obvious point: This is not a life-affirming injury. Whether we think that our old self has died or just that this new life is unimaginably hard, always think positively and never give up. The Marine officer reminds himself of this, and it helps him reaffirm why he is still here, walking this good earth:

> "Your life is God's gift to you. What you do with that life is your gift
> to God."

"Thinking positively" might sound like a cliché, but like the alcoholic or drug addict who takes it one day at a time, simple phrases of truth are hard won by survivors of all kinds. What might sound like clichés can take on enormous meaning when your life is on the line. Often, they are why we are surviving. We've thought about them so hard and applied them so vigorously that sometimes we dare to stand tall and are proud for a moment because against all odds, we believed and acted on these things: Easy does it – Live and let live – First things first – One day at a time –Keep it simple.

MOVING FROM AWARENESS TO ADJUSTMENT

This chapter has been the final slog through the most painful period of a brain injury: Awareness. With the next section, Adjustment, your soundtrack should be the William Tell Overture. Turn it up. Help is on the way.

ADJUSTMENT

"It is not the strongest of the species that survives,

nor the most intelligent that survives.

It is the one that is the most adaptable to change."

Charles Darwin

13 – Contact State BIA and/or BIAA

BEGIN BY CONTACTING YOUR STATE'S BIA

Many people with brain injuries – especially those newly diagnosed – don't know where to turn, and neither do their loved ones and caregivers. Finding the right doctor is an important step in recovery, but one too often made through trial-and-error. We can't simply Google "brain injury doctor" and expect find the right provider. The suspicion or discovery that our general physician or even many specialists can't provide answers to our questions increases our desperation and isolation. A state BIA is a good starting point. Most states have one, and at a minimum should have a website that describes its services. Most are affiliated with the Brain Injury Association of America (BIAA), for which they pay an annual membership fee.

Quality and focus vary widely from state to state

I recently joined a useful group on LinkedIn called BI-IFEA (Brain Injury – Ideas for Education & Advocacy), and provoked quite a response when I posted an open question about the quality of state BIAs.

On the plus side, one person said great things about the BIA of Minnesota. They provided her with resource coordination, contracted case worker services, a peer-mentor program, a speaker's bureau and consumer advocacy training. They offered opportunities to volunteer, raise money, and made her feel as though she was making a difference. It also prints a Consumer Guide each year that lists many providers of a wide variety of services.

Funding is always a major issue. Maine's BIA recently shut down for lack of funds. Many BIAs emphasize prevention, which is helpful for the general population but of little use to someone with a brain injury. Some associations have an army of one whose main job is to answer the phone and try to get that first interaction right. This book will help you take full advantage of the services offered to the brain-injured and their caregivers.

Madelaine Sayko

In the previous chapter I quoted Madelaine Sayko, a brain-injury advocate and educator who notes that is helpful to understand what a BIA can and can't do for you. State BIAs follow the guidelines of the Alliance of Information and Referral Systems (AIRS). AIRS directs BIAs to offer tools to find resources and, without providing direction referrals, give more than one choice. Callers might desire specific and personal recommendations, but a BIA must remain neutral to avoid even the appearance of conflict of interest.

The selection of a provider has to be a personal choice and, even without legal restrictions, a BIA can't get in the business of referring. Few general practitioners undergo formal brain-injury training to, for example, clarify the impact of a brain injury on endocrine function, or distinguish between brain injury and mental illness.

BIAs usually have a very small paid staff, a volunteer staff, and limited resources for marketing, technology and supporting complex service needs. One challenge of providing information to consumers is that it quickly becomes outdated. New agencies or organizations might be formed, others might change names or contact information, or they might fade away completely – sometimes within a single month. Because new organizations, services, treatments, processes and requirements update all the time, keeping all this current requires a dedicated team.

A brain injury association exists to provide information, educate the community at large and, when possible, provide tools to help survivors rebuild their lives after a brain injury. These are big tasks, and the needs of the brain injured are incredibly diverse. We have to be realistic. Even when a BIA cannot directly answer your question, they should be able to help you find someone who can.

While most BIAs direct a person to a medical center that has physicians specializing in brain injury – such as a neurologist or neuropsychologist – they can't accurately appraise one. Few objective measures exist that a BIA can apply to facilities, nor can a BIA ascertain the quality of care for every type of brain injury. The only basis that a BIA can use is whether a facility has the appropriate certifications, such as The Joint Commission (TJC)[11], which accredits over 19,000 health care organizations and programs in the US.

Smaller, more informal brain-injury organizations

BIAs in large states or states with many rural areas might not have access to local organizations, but they will likely know some of the bigger groups who in turn can help you regionally. These groups – whether they are support groups or care facilities – should introduce themselves to the BIA to spread word of their services. Individuals in support groups and at centers can then share their experiences and personal feedback.

Many folks with brain injury want and need a more individualized approach in traversing this journey successfully. The range of issues is vast – financial, legal, housing, technology, supports, education, social, vocational, physical and more. All of these concerns and questions require answers and insight. Here, too, informal networks, such as online communities, support groups and centers can be wonderful, rich sources for information. But by definition – "informal" – they have limits.

Support groups and on-line communities can sometimes identify who is good with what; for example, severe vs. moderate vs. mild brain injury, vocational supports, acquired versus traumatic. They also exchange experiences about particular agencies and programs, but these are informal opinions, and the amount of data can quickly become overwhelming. And always remember that opinion is opinion, and if it worked for Sally it might not work for Sue. It takes shopping around, and listening to your own gut. That is often hard for someone with a brain injury, and sometimes using an advocate to find your way through this maze is helpful.

Using an advocate

An advocate can be a family member, a good friend or someone who is paid to help you – but it is strongly recommended that you have some help. Madelaine explained to me that some states endorse the idea of having a formal patient-advocate role that you can hire either out-of-pocket or through state funding. Such an advocate would be able to help you select the best options that made sense for you. Still, state-sponsored advocates would have to be trained and certified and there is now no national program for that.

Social workers can be great TBI resources, but sometimes they are limited in what they know, especially if they are not specifically trained in brain injury. Conversely, social workers who are trained in brain injury might not be knowledgeable about the other wide-ranging issues such as food stamps, technical assistance, transportation benefits, local community services or educational grants. A helpful way to find social workers with brain injury knowledge is to contact medical centers with brain injury programs. They might be able to direct you to someone who can help.

In Chapter 16: Making the Most of Your Appointments, you will learn more about how to, well, like the title says. Having a supportive advocate is important for a variety of reasons, even if it's a friend. For example, because of our inability to process information well and to remember any of it at all, many times we begin a search for resources but then we lose track, we put our stacks of paper aside and, associating them with a painful and frustrating experience, we forget about them. And when the stubborn among us lack the self-awareness of our own deficits, someone who knows your strengths and limitations well can be a big help in improving the quality of our lives.

Advocates can set up appointments for you, and make sure you know when and where you have to be. They can also help obtain services from a variety of agencies for educational supports and vocational training. This process can be a challenge for the brain-injured to navigate and master. Because people often assume too much about a survivor's capabilities, we might not receive the individualized type of care we need. We might "present well" but have serious deficiencies that are not obvious. We can have processing struggles but still be capable of being productive, effective, creative and even organized, even if only in "bursts" of 20 or 30 minutes. Another person might do better with visual instruction than auditory, and so needs a little more time to complete a task, or they need to have things written out.

If you do not have an advocate, seek one out

If you do not have a person like this in your life, begin by seeking out such a person. Until that time, rather than divide one notebook into many sections, designate one notebook for each major category in your life: for example, Medical, Rehabilitation, Spouse, Musings, Commentary on Spousal Musings. Bring the appropriate notebook(s) with you to all appointments, and try to write down at least a few key words from everything that is said.

Some state BIAs stand out

Madelaine writes from Pennsylvania, where the BIA helps identify resources for care, provides educational materials, directs people to nearby support groups and helps complete application forms for state assistance. BIA-PA also has a program to help with school re-entry called Brain Steps, and produces events to educate the public. BIA-PA also makes its voice heard in the government, and this legislative advocacy plays an important role.

I would be remiss if I did not mention some of the work we do at the Massachusetts BIA, where I serve on the board. Here is our mission:

> BIA-MA provides support to brain injury survivors and their families, offers programs to prevent brain injuries, educates the public on the risks and impact of brain injury, and advocates for legislation and improved services.

We are especially good at serving 33 statewide support groups, "a number no other BIA chapter approaches," our President Kenneth Kolpan states proudly. What state BIAs will learn is that if they focus on the needs of brain-injury patients and their caregivers, they almost don't need an advertising budget. Don't quote me on that. In our 2010-2011 annual report, Kolpan says, "Many participants have become Ambassadors for BIA-MA, spreading its message of prevention and increasing awareness of brain injury statewide."

The state of BIAs today

Brain-injury awareness is still a very new topic. BIAs and other groups are trying to find their footing. Some states are pursuing ways to serve their brain-injured community more diligently than others. Nationwide, whether because of the NFL and NHL, or the jaw-dropping highway statistics on brain injury, an awareness of the far-reaching consequences of brain injury is growing very quickly. And when the Centers for Disease Control and Prevention (CDC) can get a handle on data that is slow to emerge from India and China, brain injury will soon have worldwide recognition as a crisis. It is currently a silent epidemic, but not for long; the brain-injured and our supporters are beginning to find our voices and raise them.

BIAs continue to grow in response to demand and resources. Those of us in the field, whether professionally involved or looking up off the ground, are hopeful that this attention will lead to more research, better understanding and education, improved treatments and more support for brain-injury associations of many kinds. They can do a lot of good, offering educational conferences and alternative sources of information. In the complex arena of brain injury they can be a very good place to begin.

Looking into your state's BIA

After receiving immediate care after your initial contacts, you might want to learn more about your state's BIA. Madelaine suggests asking them:

- What is your long-term vision? What are your short-term goals?

- Why do you seem to focus on one particular topic – say, prevention?

- Where does your funding come from?

- How many people on your staff and board have a brain injury? How many are caregivers in some way?

She goes on to suggest that you volunteer, and to encourage family and friends to do the same. This will help you learn more about what is happening with legislation and resources, and identify ways to help improve the status quo. You might find you can make a big difference in such issues as social marginalization, financial insecurities, and political under-representation.

Grass-roots alternatives

Finally, recognize that positive change is often won slowly. You will have noticed by now that you have to take many matters into your own hands. If you still believe that your state's BIA is not providing you with what you need, seek out or form a grass-roots group that will. Small grass-roots groups are free to focus their effort and attentions on specific issues, such as socialization or teens with brain injury.

Grass-roots groups can fill in the more specific gaps and needs of an area, as do the Brain Injury Alliance in Colorado and the BI Resource Center in Wisconsin. Madelaine volunteers with her BIA but she also serves on a board of a local group: Acquired Brain Injury Network Of Pennsylvania, Inc. (ABIN-PA). ABIN-PA is very community based and does a lot of peer-to-peer work directly with survivors. They also reach out to local organizations – police, group homes, EMTs, and mental health agencies – to educate them on brain injury behaviors and symptoms. They are well-regarded, have a strong presence in the Harrisburg area, and co-ordinate their efforts with the BIA-PA.

IF YOU ARE NOT SATISFIED, CONTACT THE BIAA

About the Brain Injury Association of America

If you live in one of the states that do not have one, or if you are not satisfied with the services your state's BIA provides, contact the BIAA at 800-444-6443 or through www.biausa.org and they will help you. For example, the BIAA is helpful if you believe that your state's association does not have up-to-date information about the latest imaging technology. The BIAA stays current on the most advanced technologies in the brain-injury world, although they would be the first to tell you that far more medical research and technological advances are needed.

Founded in 1980, the BIAA is the leading national organization serving and representing individuals, families and professionals who are affected by a traumatic brain injury. Together with its network of more than 40 chartered state affiliates, as well as hundreds of local chapters and support groups across the country, the BIAA provides information, education and support to assist the more than three million Americans currently living with TBI, as well as their families.

The national office is very good at helping people find resources in states that have no BIA presence. They are good at this because, as one BIAA director told me, "We have to be." He said they can at least identify programs with brain-injury expertise and they know how to quickly find resources, such as Case Managers or neuropsychologists.

FINDING AN ATTENDING PHYSICIAN AND A CASE MANAGER

So, either from your state's BIA or the BIAA, ask for help finding two critical resources who will guide your recovery:

- An Attending Physician

- A Neurotrauma Rehabilitation Specialist, who can function as your Case Manager

Your state's BIA should have its finger on the pulse of local TBI resources. The BIAA, on the other hand, does not keep a list of neurologists that specialize in brain-injury rehabilitation, and will suggest you contact the American Academy of Neurology at www.aan.com. As a BIAA Director told me:

> The biggest challenge is to find professionals with expertise in brain injury, and to find the right professional.

1. Attending Physician

Your Attending Physician might be a neurologist, a D.O. (Doctor of Osteopathy), or a physiatrist (a medical doctor specializing in physical medicine and rehabilitation), but should have experience working with TBI patients.

My Attending Physician happens to be a D.O.

You might decide to choose a D.O. to be your Attending Physician. Like an M.D. a D.O. is a fully licensed physician who can practice in any specialty, such as pediatrics, internal medicine, psychiatry, surgery, or obstetrics. Most are General Practitioners. Unlike an M.D., an osteopath approaches her practice from a more holistic perspective.

She treats your body as a unity, emphasizing "wellness" and identifying specific ways that preventive medicine can contribute to your total health in relation to the risks associated with your particular stresses at home and at work. She also evaluates the muscular-skeletal system to manage pain or other difficulties caused by traumatic brain injury.

Neurologist

Neurology is a medical specialty that focuses on the disorders and pathologies of the nervous system – the brain, nerves, spinal cord and associated muscle and tissue. Neurologists are medical doctors who have completed a year of training in internal medicine plus a three-year residency in neurology. Some neurologists have additional training in a specialty such as sleep disorder, epilepsy, or the management of pain; others are clinical researchers.

Neurologists are trained to perform and evaluate tests such as the CT scan, MRI and EEG. If you were sent to an emergency room after your trauma, a neurologist probably ordered and evaluated your tests.

If you have mild TBI and are referred, as I was, to a *neurosurgeon* you might find that they especially will be at a loss for what to do with you. Neurosurgeons know how to cut skulls open, take out tumors, relieve pressure or whatever, and then, because it's in their job descriptions, they can put your brains and skull back together again. But even neurosurgeons cannot know everything, even when it comes to recovering from a brain injury. This is why typically they hand off TBI patients to one or more specialists, as described in Chapter 15 – Building Your Recovery Team: REHABILITATION.

Whether you are contacting a neurologist or a D.O., be sure to ask how much experience she has working with brain-injured patients. A Director at BIAA told me:

> You may find a neurologist to be really helpful in dealing with a specific issue post-injury (like headaches or pain) but they are not helpful in dealing with cognitive and emotional issues post-injury.

These post-injury issues can best be addressed with the help of a Case Manager, sometimes called a Neurotrauma Rehabilitation Specialist.

2. Neurotrauma Rehabilitation Specialist

The second person to contact is a neurotrauma rehabilitation specialist. My Case Manager Beth Adams told me she invented the term some years ago, so a formal definition or description of the neurotrauma rehabilitation discipline is a bit of a moving target. A prominent medical center professor and director told me that there is no formal certification in "cognitive neuro-trauma rehabilitation," but that clinicians with specialty training and experience in this area can come from a range of interdisciplinary backgrounds.

This specialist or counselor can be a clinician licensed to practice in any number of disciplines, such as occupational therapy, neuropsychology or speech-language pathology. Any of the recovery team members included in the next chapter might legitimately present themselves as neurotrauma rehabilitation specialists provided they have significant experience working with the kind of brain injury you have, whether mild or severe.

A neurotrauma rehab specialist has additional training and experience in evaluating and treating patients with a brain dysfunction acquired from an injury or illness that has compromised how the survivor thinks and feels.

Your neurotrauma rehab specialist will have board certification or a license in her particular area of expertise, but you need to confirm that she has experience working with the brain injured. Ask her something like, "How long have you been treating people with TBI?" While no objective measurement exists for a qualified specialist, a professional with multiple years of practice in the field, working with TBI survivors, should be the most effective working with you in your recovery.

Case manager as quarterback

I think of Beth Adams as a quarterback and I'm the football because she makes sure I'm in the right hands. A Licensed Rehabilitation Counselor (M. Ed. LRC) and speech therapist, she has more than 25 years of experience in the brain injury field. If I have a question, Beth generally has the answer; when she doesn't, she always puts me in touch with the person who does.

Because of her vast experience, Beth helped me understand what had happened to me and put me in touch with every member of my recovery team:

> I work in multiple areas to help the patient. I have a speech-language background, but because of my experience I know that people with a brain injury can easily fall through the cracks of the medical system. I know where the holes are in the brain injury world so people don't have to fall into an abyss. Helping them navigate the system is essential toward the road to recovery.

The mother of a teenage daughter came to Beth three years into her daughter's injury. Both mother and daughter were lost, frustrated and afraid, just as I was after my injury. This woman put it this way: "Before we met Beth we were hamsters on a wheel. When we met Beth, the wheel stopped." They started getting the help they needed.

(<u>Note</u>: Be sure to inquire whether your health plan covers Case Manager services. Many plans will not, and you have to weigh that cost carefully.)

Ideal outcomes

I believe this list describes ideal outcomes for your first meetings with your Attending Physician and Case Manager:

- In your first meeting with your Attending Physician and your Case Manager, they ask about your incident and you describe your sequelae.

- They listen attentively, take notes, and then say, "You appear to have a textbook case of a traumatic brain injury."

- If you have a so-called mild TBI, they explain that your incident caused stretching and tearing at the neuron level. Your injury doesn't show up on your CT scan, MRI, or EEG because mild TBI rarely does, but it's real nonetheless. Your injury has caused the effects you've described and has devastated you.

- Having heard this you're still frightened, but you also feel enormous relief. You think, "Finally, somebody gets it." All of this horrible stuff you've been experiencing – it's the result of your head injury, and it's real. You're not crazy after all.

You feel reassured: At last somebody has put a name to your mysterious ailment. Yet this so-called mild TBI has wrecked you. What do you do next? Who can help you? The answer is: your recovery team.

DESIGN A RECOVERY TEAM THAT MEETS YOUR NEEDS

Your Attending Physician and Case Manager should see to it that you begin working with the appropriate resources. You will then work with two sets of specialists in your recovery:

- <u>MEDICAL</u>: Attending Physician refers you to medical resources

- <u>REHABILITATION</u>: Case Manager refers you to various therapies

Although many sequelae might overlap, every brain injury is different. It follows that your recovery team might differ from mine. For instance, my injury left me with some significant cognitive challenges, so I worked very closely with experienced speech-language pathologist Rick Sanders. If your injury left you with serious physical challenges, you should see a physical therapist. If your sequelae are keeping you from working, you should ask to be referred to a good vocational rehab specialist.

Again, make sure that each team member has experience with your level of TBI, whether it is mild, moderate, or severe.

14 – Building Your Recovery Team: MEDICAL

OVERVIEW

Your Attending Physician refers you to other doctors as necessary. But, especially when we are new to our injury, the most accurate way to describe how we are feeling to an Attending Physician is, "I feel awful." "Awful" or "terrible" could mean any number of things, or any combination of things. These simple descriptors don't give the doctor much to go on, even if he (or she) has a lot of experience working with TBI patients.

In the doctor's mind should be a checklist of specialists to gradually work down. Here is a list of some of the medical specialists you might need to see:

Figure 5:

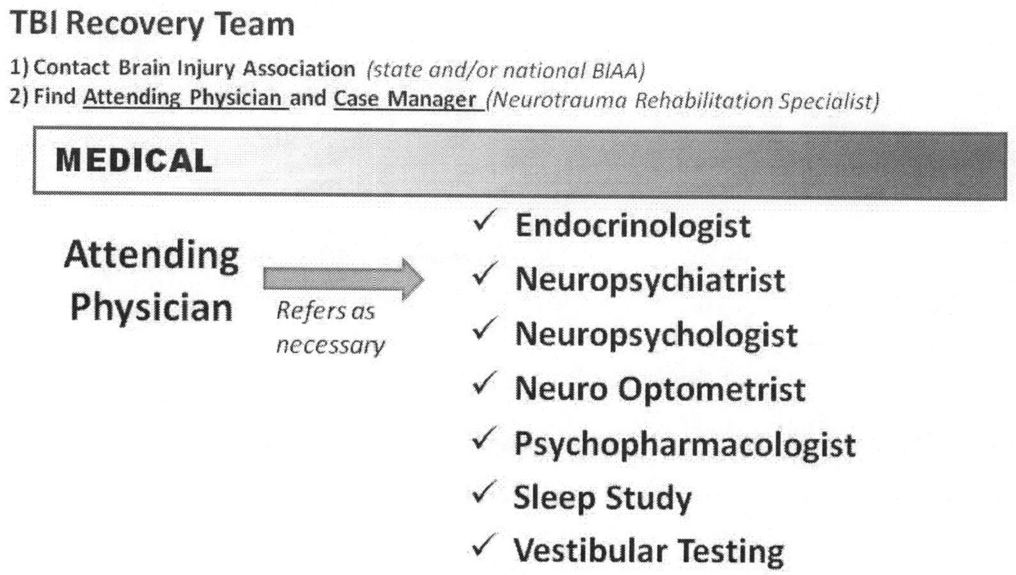

TBI Recovery Team

1) Contact Brain Injury Association *(state and/or national BIAA)*
2) Find <u>Attending Physician</u> and <u>Case Manager</u> *(Neurotrauma Rehabilitation Specialist)*

MEDICAL

Attending Physician → *Refers as necessary*

✓ **Endocrinologist**
✓ **Neuropsychiatrist**
✓ **Neuropsychologist**
✓ **Neuro Optometrist**
✓ **Psychopharmacologist**
✓ **Sleep Study**
✓ **Vestibular Testing**

ENDOCRINOLOGIST

What might "feeling awful" mean?

I know a survivor who felt deeply fatigued and depressed for five years before his neurologist suggested that he see an endocrinologist and get a complete workup. This was a guy whose MRI had been looked at by a number of neurologists who deemed it "clean" because they could see no obvious bleeding or bruising to the brain. The endocrinologist, however, slapped the same MRI up on the lightbox, took one look at the pituitary gland and said, "I don't like the looks of that."

After ordering a new, more intensive MRI (this one took 45 minutes), the endocrinologist took a closer look at the pituitary gland and diagnosed empty sella syndrome (ESS). He explained that the bony structure at the base of the brain that protects the pituitary gland is called the sella turcica. Sometimes, radiological imaging of the pituitary gland reveals a sella turcica that appears to be empty ("partially empty sella"). This often results in abnormal levels of testosterone and human growth hormone, and the patient needs to receive supplemental doses of one or both.

Feeling awful might well be because your endocrinology system is out of whack. The endocrine system, through the secretion of hormones, regulates virtually every activity in the human body and TBI can cause it to go haywire. In fact, studies indicate that:

- Many TBI patients have some form of endocrine dysfunction.

- Roughly 40 percent of people with TBI have hypopituitarism, which is the underproduction of hormones.[12]

According to Endotext, "the most accessed source on endocrinology for Medical Professionals":

> Abnormal axes during the acute phase of injury may recover over time, but other pituitary hormone deficits may evolve later even at six months after the initial insult.
>
> . . . it has been suggested that patients with TBI should be assessed on presentation and at six months post injury. [13]

At least initially, an endocrinologist should be on your recovery team. Ask your doctor to refer you to one for a complete endocrinology workup. Not all endocrinologists are familiar with the impact a TBI can have on the endocrine system. Make sure that the endocrinologist knows about your incident and that you might have a brain injury. Your test results should be analyzed with that in mind.

Mike's endocrinology numbers

As with acceptable cholesterol or blood pressure numbers, endocrine numbers are a gauge. For example, a male without a TBI between the ages of 18-65 generally has testosterone numbers ranging from 200 to 1100. After Mike's brain injury his numbers dropped way below the bottom of that range, and he felt terrible all the time. He lost his libido, couldn't sleep, had very little energy, and had severe problems with his speech. His endocrinologist prescribed the maximum amount of a testosterone replacement therapy, but it didn't budge Mike's numbers.

Figure 6:

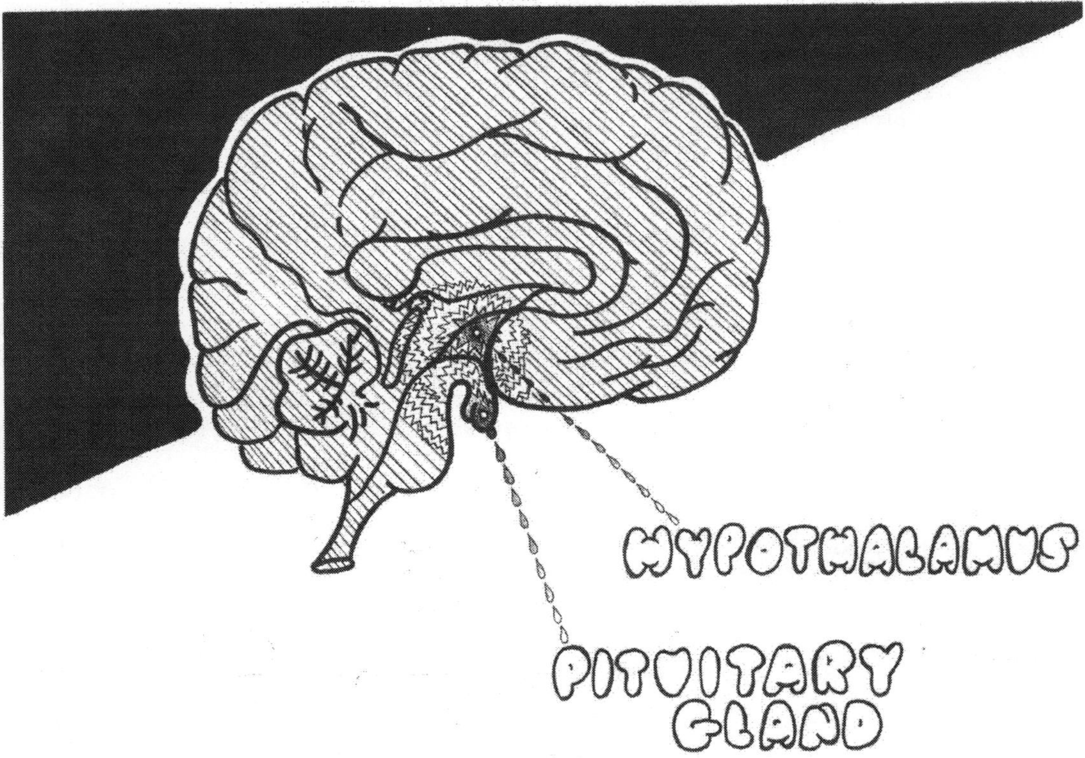

<u>*Artwork*</u>: *Chris Byler*

Mike started researching the connection between TBI and endocrinology. He made an appointment with an endocrinologist who is a leading expert on the relationship between endocrine numbers and TBI. His previous endocrinologist had told Mike that if they could bump his testosterone numbers up to 400, he'd feel better. The new specialist explained that, in his opinion, 400 for Mike was not acceptable, and that for a man with TBI, the numbers should be in the top 25 percent range of "normal."

He then prescribed high doses of testosterone to bring Mike's numbers up to 800 and the treatment is making a significant difference. Before his treatments

Mike says he was "comatose." The ongoing treatments have corrected his libido and energy levels, elevated his mood, helped his speech, enabled him to sleep better, and even helped him to socialize a little easier with people.

There are downsides. Some people have the misconception that testosterone supplements cause cancer. They don't cause cancer, but they can cause cancer to spread more quickly. Also, these treatments are expensive, and might not be covered by your insurer.

<u>Note</u>: Appendix F provides a brief but informative question-and-answer session with Mike.

The Hormone Foundation

A helpful place to turn is The Hormone Foundation[14], the public education affiliate of The Endocrine Society. It is a leading source of hormone-related health information for the public, physicians, allied health professionals and the media. Its mission is to "serve as a resource for the public by promoting the prevention, treatment and cure of hormone-related conditions through outreach and education."

NEUROPSYCHIATRIST

In my fourth year of recovery, my D.O. referred me to a doctor at Massachusetts General Hospital and I said, "Great. I will see anyone you suggest, any time." When I called to make the appointment the voice on the line answered, "Psychiatry."

"Psychiatry"? The word twisted my insides. Was my D.O. suggesting – did he believe – that the array of cognitive and emotional problems I had been wrestling with were psychiatric in nature or origin? In that instant I felt a rush of emotions: confusion, anger, frustration, loneliness, sadness and even despair. I made the appointment anyway, making good on my commitment to see anyone he suggested.

I arrived in Boston that day with an open mind, determined to place myself in whatever hands might be healing hands. The doctor turned out to be a neuropsychiatrist, which is a different kettle of fish. I felt enormous relief: a neuropsychiatrist was going to evaluate my clinical cognitive problems, not those garden-variety psychological problems.

He spent 90 minutes with me, a big chunk of time for a doctor to commit to one patient. He asked me to talk about my accident, and the first days and weeks after the accident. He asked for details about my sequelae and my bad experiences with various medications. He assured me that if I preferred, we could take a therapeutic route other than a psychopharmacological one. Throughout he listened attentively, focusing totally on my descriptions of my injury.

Then he said something I had been waiting and strangely enough even longing to hear from a doctor during my so-called recovery: "Everything you've described is consistent with mild TBI." He set me at ease because of his professional demeanor, and I felt enormous confidence in him when he told me that all his patients are survivors of mild TBI. I knew I was finally in the right hands.

Neuropsychiatry is a very new field

Until a few years ago it was impossible to get a neurologist and a psychiatrist in the same room together. My friend David (Chapter 6) can tell you that from firsthand experience.

Shortly after his injury David was seeing both a neurologist, who took him off medication for his bi-polar disorder, and a psychiatrist. The psychiatrist said that he was angry the neurologist had taken David off his meds and told him to come back only when he was back on them. David asked both doctors to meet with him at the same time and they refused. "I could not understand separating the 'brain' from the 'mind,'" David recalls. "When I was in New York in the 1970s, I got to know a neurologist at Columbia Presbyterian. He told me the faculty at Johns Hopkins would not allow him to study both fields."

In the last ten years or so, the adversarial relationship of the two disciplines ended with the emergence of neuropsychiatry. According to Neurotrauma Registry:

> Neuropsychiatry is the medical specialty committed to better understanding brain-behavior relationships, and to the care of individuals with neurologically based cognitive, emotional, and behavioral disturbances.
>
> What is a neuropsychiatrist? A neuropsychiatrist is a physician (M.D. or D.O.) qualified to practice neuropsychiatry by virtue of either:
>
> 1. Primary training in either psychiatry or neurology followed by at least one year of fellowship training in neuropsychiatry/behavioral neurology, or

2. Formal residency training in both neurology and psychiatry. Psychiatrists or neurologists with many years of extensive clinical, educational and scientific experience in the field of neuropsychiatry may also merit this special designation.

The two disciplines were divided because neurology "focused objectively on organic nervous system pathology ('inside-the-skin' perspective), especially of the brain, whereas psychiatrists have laid claim to illnesses of the mind ('outside-the-skin' causation – personal, interpersonal, cultural)." Academic clinicians began to see this distinction as contrived.[15]

Dr. Joseph B. Martin, a neurology professor and Dean of Harvard Medical School, argued for an alliance between the two fields. In 2002 he wrote:

The separation of the two categories is arbitrary, often influenced by beliefs rather than proven scientific observations. And the fact that the brain and mind are one makes the separation artificial anyway. [16]

Why separate neurology and psychiatry?

As I said, David puzzled over the separation more than 20 years ago when he was injured: "Why would anybody separate the brain from the mind?" The emergence of neuropsychiatry reflects the idea that "brain and mind are not discrete entities but just different ways of looking at the same system."

Even if your neuropsychiatrist does not specifically diagnose you with TBI, mild or otherwise, she can help you address your cognitive, physical and emotional/behavioral problems through drug therapies and/or behavioral therapies.

NEUROPSYCHOLOGIST

If you've got mild TBI, you're likely to face a one-two punch. The first punch is that conventional diagnostic tests – CT scans, PET scans, MRIs and EEGs – do not detect the stretching, tearing and twisting of the neurons in the brain that leave lasting damage. The second is more of a psychic punch: You look normal, so everybody thinks you are normal. Your injury is invisible to everyone but you.

Consider the mild TBI survivors who remain undiagnosed, whose suffering has not been validated by medical professionals. All they know is that "something's wrong" and they "feel different." Suddenly they have trouble with short-term memory or find it difficult to concentrate or they have suffocating anxiety attacks. These survivors might feel mostly relief that they're alive and so anything short of death seems too trivial to raise with a doctor or family. But the sequelae will not go away – they will wear you down until they dominate your whole life, and eventually sap the life from you.

So let's say that your doctor has informed you that your MRI is normal, but your boss calls you into his office and says, "Why is the quality of your work so poor these days? Is everything okay? I mean, you look fine, so what's the problem?" Or let's say a year after your injury the jurors deliberating on your case keep circling back to your normal appearance and your normal CT scan. They scratch their heads and ask one another, "Why should we award him damages?"

Neuropsych testing: "invisible injury" doesn't mean it's unquantifiable

Enter your neuropsychologist who has training and experience in choosing, administering, and interpreting sophisticated diagnostic tests that are designed to identify and assess brain function deficits. In some cases, they can also help you identify the incident that might have caused your injury.

This person is a core member of your recovery team. From these tests, usually conducted over a series of two or three days because of your reduced stamina, they can diagnose you, and facilitate your rehabilitation.

If your injury involves a lawsuit, they can provide critical forensic evidence of your injury in a courtroom. On his website Brainsource.com, neuropsychologist Dennis P. Swiercinsky writes:

> While neurological examination and CT, MRI, EEG and PET scans look at the structural, physical and metabolic condition of the brain, the neuropsychological examination is the only way to formally assess brain function.
>
> Neuropsychological tests cover the range of mental processes from simple motor performance to complex reasoning and problem solving. In almost all objective tests, quantitative results are compared with some normative standard, including data from groups of non-brain injured persons and groups of persons with various kinds of brain injury…
>
> The combination of objective scores, behavioral process observations, and consistency in emerging pattern of results, along with comprehensive clinical history, constitute the art and science of neuropsychological assessment. [17]

Examples

Here are three randomly selected examples included in a list of over 70 tests[18]:

Boston Naming Test	Assessing the ability to name pictures of objects through spontaneous responses and need for various types of cueing. Inferences can be drawn regarding language facility and possible localization of cerebral damage.
MicroCog	This computerized assessment measures nine functional cognitive areas sensitive to brain injury
Grooved Pegboard	This procedure measures performance speed in a fine motor task. By examining both sides of the body, inferences may be drawn regarding possible lateral brain damage.

Examples from my testing

The neuropsych exam I took included these activities:

- Seeing a series of faces in a flipbook and then identifying which appeared and did not appear in a second series.

- Having a minute to think of as many words as I could that start with the letter "a," and then repeating the test for the letter "s."

- Having a minute to think of as many boys' names as I could.

- Having a minute to alternate fruit and furniture ("lemon" "table" "apple" "desk").

- He placed six blue blocks in front of me. I was supposed to retrace his steps as he randomly touched four of them; we repeated the process for five, then six blocks. Then we did all of this with me retracing his steps backwards.

- Completing two pages of basic math.

- Restating a series of numbers forwards then backwards.

- Pairing up random letters and numbers in ascending order; so "L 2 O 7 1 B" would become "1 2 7 B L O".

- Answering basic history questions, such as identifying Gandhi, Martin Luther King Jr., Cleopatra and Marie Curie.

- Answering short civics questions, such as "Why do we pay taxes?" and "What is government for?"

- Re-drawing from memory an elaborate drawing of a shape, first right away and then about a half-hour later.

- Explaining how two things are alike, such as "eggs and seeds" and "monarchy and democracy."

- Identifying what should be the fifth shape when seeing pictures of sets of four increasingly complex shapes.

- Restating as much as I could remember from two paragraphs read aloud to me.

- Restating 16 random objects read aloud to me. He did this five times until I got them all right. (For the record, as long as I'm recording these things: cabinet, bookcase, desk, lamp, truck, motorcycle, subway, boat, squirrel, cow, giraffe, zebra, onion, celery, cabbage, spinach.)

A week or so later, he mailed me a detailed summary of my results. He then called to debrief them with Lynne and me. He explained that he compared my percentiles with the general population of men of my demographic. While some of my results were in the superior range, he said that "efficiency of processing is the problem, relative to the baseline," meaning it took me longer compared with other people like me before my injury.

Intact intellect does not mean a lack of a brain injury

Having a brain injury does not always mean a degrading of intellect. I do have a close friend who has suffered from epileptic seizures all his life, and over the years has, as he put it, "lost entire shelves of Latin and Hebrew." But especially with a mild TBI, even your vocabulary and memory of books read and insights learned can be intact. Again, the injury shows itself in things like processing speed, fluency, word retrieval and sheer intellectual stamina.

Heads up, the tests are exhausting!

My friend Elizabeth describes her experience:

> Big 24 hours for this gal...holy moly, I'm exhausted! Had a neuropsych exam today; glad it's out of the way. It was really bizarre. I feel like there were times when I blatantly didn't know what was going on or I felt like I was acing it. No idea what they're going to say about it all, or how they would interpret a test like that!! Really interesting though.
>
> It absolutely EXHAUSTED me. I couldn't even keep my eyes open for a whole section! I know I had a hard time with one part where they showed me pictures and asked me what's missing. I could never find anything!
>
> Makes sense, though. That's one thing I've struggled with a lot – attention to detail.

Critical piece of puzzle

Neuropsychologist tests are a critical piece of the puzzle, helping to identify, describe, and objectively evaluate the damage to your brain and, as attorney Kenneth Kolpan puts it, your "isles of competence." Informed by the test results, you can focus on the therapies that can speed your rehabilitation and allow you to work more effectively with other specialists on your recovery team.

NEURO-OPTOMETRIST

One of the most common sequelae survivors tell me about is their change in vision after the injury. Sometimes one eye's vision is blurry, forcing the other eye to work harder, which can lead to terrible headaches. One survivor spent two hours with someone she had been told was an excellent neuro-optometrist, only to "learn" that he could not find anything wrong with her vision. He had made no attempt to link her new vision problems with her brain injury, nor did he explain why she could not see straight and suffered migraines.

But, as with most of the information in this book, don't take my word for it. Even a quick look at the Neuro-Optometric Rehabilitation Association website reveals an estimate that 80 to 85 percent "of our perception, learning, cognition and activities are mediated through vision. The ultimate purpose of the visual process is to arrive at an appropriate motor, and/or cognitive response."[19] It would make sense, then, that a TBI, mild or more severe, might negatively affect one's vision, and that one's vision might affect the sequelae of the injury.

In fact, the same website states that more than 50 percent of neurologically impaired patients – such as TBI and MS – experience visual and visual-cognitive disorders. More specifically,

> "Visual-perceptual dysfunction is one of the most common devastating residual impairments of head injury." Barbara Zoltan, M.A., O.T.R. [20]

Clearly, finding the right neuro-optometrist is critical if you are suffering from this dysfunction. For more information, go to the Neuro-Optometric Rehabilitation Association website at http://www.nora.cc/

PSYCHOPHARMACOLOGIST

Your psychopharmacologist prescribes medications that can alleviate some of the sequelae you are experiencing, such as depression and anxiety, lability, sleep disorders, and cognitive problems. While you should be cautious of hasty prescriptions, try not to be prejudiced either for or against medications because the injury might have affected your brain's chemistry. The proper medication might be the one part of your therapy that helps the most.

It could also be extremely uncomfortable until you and your psychopharmacologist determine the best fit for you. While the process is not exactly hit or miss, it can sometimes feel that way. One med might be prescribed in increasing dosages and you might find, as I did with Namenda, that all of your sequelae get worse. But if you and your psychopharmacologist can be patient, you might be able to find the med or meds that are just right for you. (Being patient is one thing, but having "suicidal ideations" is another, of course. It is intolerable to have your already miserable day-to-day experience get worse. Speak up immediately about how you react to a med.)

What is psychopharmacology, exactly? The American Society of Clinical Psychopharmacology (ASCP) defines it as the:

> . . . study of the use of medications in treating mental disorders . . . Psychopharmacologists need to understand all the clinically relevant

principles of pharmacokinetics (what the body does to medication) and pharmacodynamics (what the medications do to the body).

Since the use of these medications is to treat mental disorders, an extensive understanding of basic neuroscience, basic psychopharmacology, clinical medicine, the differential diagnosis of mental disorders, and treatment options is required. [21]

According to the ASCP "any physician who treats patients with psychotropic medication is a psychopharmacologist." This means that when your neuropsychiatrist or your neurologist prescribes a medication to alleviate your sleep difficulties, this person is acting as a psychopharmacologist. Any doctor who has completed residency training after medical school has pharmacological expertise. Psychiatrists, who train an additional four years after medical school, have more sophisticated expertise in psychopharmacology.

You might decide to see a doctor who specializes in psychopharmacology: that is, a doctor trained in advanced psychopharmacology in an academic institution, or through Continuing Medical Education (CME), or self-study. The ASCP evaluates candidates through an exacting examination process that tests the physician's expertise in "all areas" of Advanced Psychopharmacology and "requires a thorough understanding of the latest science that has relevance to clinical practice."

Psychopharmacology is so nuanced, and changes in therapies can be so rapid, complex and far-reaching, that in order to keep up with the newest developments in the field, your psychopharmacologist has to take a new exam every five years.

My delicate balance

I mentioned my disastrous experience with Namenda. Other survivors find that it helps them in some way, perhaps with cognitive skills or stamina. After several years of trying, discarding and re-trying certain meds, my current pharmacological regime is as follows:

Morning: 5 mg Ritalin, 5 mg Buspar, 1000 mg Ceraxon

I described my initial experience with Ritalin and then Concerta (a time-release Methylphenidate) in Chapter 8: "Look, I'm not Phineas Gage!" but, briefly, I have learned that a small dose of Ritalin – 5 mg – helps me begin my day. It is no stronger than a cup of coffee. After maybe 5 hours it is completely out of my system and I can rest, even sleep, to recharge my cognitive battery so that I can confront the remains of the day.

Buspar (buspirone) has been prescribed to help deal with a pretty horrible feeling deep down in my gut that might be called anxiety or tension, and sometimes it feels like intense nausea. As of this writing I have been on it for only a month but I believe it is helping.

Ceraxon is the other indispensable part of my intake. One of my doctors investigated the use of citicoline for TBI patients, and asked me to consider taking half-doses of Ceraxon, a citicoline sodium supplement. Intended primary for stroke and Alzheimer's patients, this over-the-counter treatment purports to actually rebuild neurons.

As stated on www.ceraxon.com:

> "Citicoline is an essential building block and main component of all cell walls. Citicoline is also vital to the formation of acetylcholine, one of the brain's major neurotransmitters."

> "CerAxon has proven to promote rapid cell membrane repair and restore its integrity, which keeps its functions intact."

This doctor assured me good-naturedly that he has no connection with Ferrer, the manufacturer. Buying citicoline sodium online might be cheaper but he warned that the amounts vary wildly. One capsule might contain 150 mg and another capsule in the same bottle might contain 50 mg.

Because I believed I might have experienced some cognitive improvements, he had me double the amount to the recommended dosage: 2000 mg a day. We tested that amount for some number of months, I forget how many, and we have stabilized my daily intake to 1000 mg.

One piece of anecdotal evidence I can tell you is that a survivor I know from support group absolutely swears by it. She experienced vast improvements in her mood and concentration, speaking about Ceraxon in such glowing and specific terms that I was in no position to voice concerns about other possible factors playing into those improvements because, clearly, she had considered all of that. Her eyes were so filled with life when she told me how dead she had felt before.

Looking back on that conversation I'm reminded of my Facebook post after feeling frustrated when a doctor discounted my enthusiasm over a holistic treatment I had tried and liked very much. He said that no data supported such a conclusion. Mulling that over for much of the day, stewing actually, I posted, "I EXIST, THEREFORE I AM DATA."

Noon-ish: 5 or 10 mg Ritalin, 5 mg Buspar

After my mid-day rest, absolutely essential to getting through the day, I then decide whether 5 or 10 mg of Ritalin will help me get through the rest of it. This decision is a subjective one, sure, but we adults have to make these kinds of decisions all the time, don't we. I will say that I am more inclined to take the lower dose because, although I feel I can get more accomplished with 10 mg, I do pay a price with the higher dose. If you are working on a physical task you might complete it faster – more exuberantly, if you will – but you might crash harder. If you are working on a mental task, your brain has information that you might believe you need to retrieve more quickly or easily. Ritalin does not create what is not there, but I believe that only Ritalin will help me access it.

So this is my word of caution: if you imagine your brain as a sponge and information is water, Ritalin squeezes your brain to get the water out. Afterwards – even if you are happy with the result – your brain might feel as though it has been wrung dry. So, decide whether 'tis better to have extracted the information – writing this book, for example – and suffer the consequences, or never to have extracted the information at all.

Bedtime: 40 mg Celexa, 10 mg Aricept

I talked a bit about trying Celexa (citalopram) early in my injury in Chapter 12: "Loss of Self, and Depression." It helped me not only with lability – I no longer burst into tears, which obviously helps in social situations – but moving up from 20 to 40 mg has helped ease my depression. I take it every night before going to bed, which I'm told is the best time to take it because it can make you drowsy or otherwise affect alertness. There will be driving of cars in bed!

Aricept (donepezil) is a new member of the team. It is kind of sobering for me to know that my 82-year-old mother in Kansas takes Aricept to help restore her brain circuitry after a series of very small strokes she suffered when they lived in the mile-high city of Denver. In fact, stroke and Alzheimer's patients were Aricept's intended audience, I believe, but recently more and more TBI patients are finding 5 mg beneficial. My doctor has told me he has no intention of increasing the dose to 10 mg, which is the recommended dosage for many patients.

Not to be reductive about it, but I think it makes me smarter. It's hard to quantify that, I know, but shortly after taking it I found myself immersed in some college financial-aid application forms – a daunting task for anyone – and I found myself plowing through it with better concentration and stamina. Again, there might have been other factors at play, facing an overdue deadline, for example, but I did feel as though it went more smoothly than before the Aricept.

Lynne has also noticed that I can now listen to low-volume music while doing a manual task, such as putting dishes away or walking around the track. Music, in fact, both listening and playing, is taking – resuming – a more prominent place in my life, a really refreshing improvement for me. Find and file everything you can under "Improve the Quality of My Life."

Build a "therapeutic alliance" to meet your brain's unique needs

If you decide to include a psychopharmacologist on your team, be absolutely sure that she has experience with TBI survivors. Ask her to credibly cite patients who have been helped or not helped by particular meds.

Doctors can't fully understand your unique brain chemistry. What they do know is that some meds help some people, but they can't determine what will help you unless you are willing to work with them and try things. It's accurate to say that it's a hit or miss approach. This can be a very uncomfortable process because the way you find out if a med is right for you is to ramp up on it. Doctors sometimes call this ramping up process "loading up."

For example, you might have to take 5 mg for three days, 10 mg for three days after that, 15 mg and so on until you and your doctor agree on the effective dose. This is why the ASCP makes the point that "psychopharmacologists also must be skilled in building and utilizing a therapeutic alliance with the patient."[22]

For more information, go to the American Society of Clinical Psychopharmacology site at www.ascpp.org.

SLEEP STUDY

Many survivors cite sleeping as one of their biggest issues; either they are sleeping too much or too little. I slept a lot early on in the injury, and I still have major two-hour crashes every day, and more if I've had a lot of cognitive exertion. More troublesome is lack of sleep. Survivor friends have told me about the agony of sleeping only an hour or two a night, which frays their raw nerves even further.

It turns out that between 40 and 65 percent of survivors suffer from insomnia. This is really important to note because "sleeping problems may exacerbate other brain injury symptoms such as headache, emotional distress and cognitive impairment, making the rehabilitation process much harder."[23]

One reason for the insomnia is that people with brain injuries might produce low amounts of melatonin, which "regulates biological rhythms, including sleep."[24] Your doctor might suggest you try taking supplemental melatonin to see if that helps.

David and Mike

My friend David, introduced in Chapter 6, has made great strides in his recovery from a 1996 brain injury, but he is perpetually sleep deprived. And before Mike's endocrinology work-up, he suffered ghastly sleep problems:

> I have been in the dumps lately averaging about two hours of sleep a
> night. I got less than an hour last night and the night before. I am
> so drained and exhausted I can't even go for a sleep exam…I haven't
> been able to shake the exhaustion for a few weeks…I truly feel
> disabled.

A practicing physician when she sustained a severe TBI in a bicycle accident, Claudia L. Osborn wrote *Over My Head: A Doctor's Own Story of Head Injury from the Inside Looking Out*, a book widely read in TBI circles. As severe as her injury was, she did not suffer from sleep disorders. "Here's what I don't get," David remarked about Claudia. "She wanted to sleep and sleep, and you want to sleep and sleep, but I couldn't sleep if I tried!"

Apnea and C-Paps

Whatever your sleep disorder, your first step should be simply to have your primary doctor refer you for a sleep study. The study might show that you have apnea on top of your TBI, which would prevent you from sleeping deeply and benefiting from REM (rapid eye movement) stages of sleep. Apnea wakes you up throughout the night without you recalling it, wrecking what should be a sound night's sleep.

If you are diagnosed with apnea – also known as obstructive sleep apnea (OSA) – you will likely be issued a C-Pap (positive airway pressure), which will help you get a good night's sleep. The machine gently blows air through the nostrils, helping you to breathe without interruption. Studies show that three months of using a C-Pap dramatically reduced OSA in people with a brain injury.[25]

Because you have a brain injury, however, a good night's sleep will take you only so far in your recovery. It will help you to feel better but you will still drag your injury around with you the next day:

> . . . however, there was no demonstrable improvement in measures of daytime sleepiness. Participants experienced no significant changes in measures of mood, quality of life and cognitive performance after treatment for a sleep disorder. [26]

Work with your Attending Physician on your TBI-related sleep disorder. Solving the problem is a critical part of your recovery.

VESTIBULAR TESTING

To continue piecing together the puzzle that is your TBI, have your Attending Physician determine whether to refer you for vestibular testing. The three main vestibular problems you might experience as a result of your brain injury are imbalance, dizziness and vertigo.

You will remember my friend Gregg the fireman, whose injury prevents him from climbing a ladder. He went in for a full battery of vestibular testing and the results helped his doctor pinpoint his treatment.

Even a cursory Googling of "TBI Vestibular Disorders" will yield enormous amounts of information. For example, from a 1999 issue of *Neurology Report*, I learned that:

> Survivors often experience double and blurry vision, movement in their field of vision, vertigo, dizziness, involuntary eye movement, loss of hearing, and even hallucinations.
>
> These sequelae occur within a week to ten days after the incident of injury. Although most cases resolve after three months, 15 percent have persistent symptoms a whole year later. [27]

As with most aspects of recovery from a brain injury, much more work is needed in the field of TBI-related vestibular disorders. One major study concluded:

> Physical therapists are calling for definitive vestibular screenings and assessment measures for US military service members with blast-induced traumatic brain injuries (BITBI) . . . vestibular rehabilitation must be included as part of successful treatment for those who have been injured by blasts and experience vestibular symptoms such as vertigo, gaze instability and motion intolerance. [28]

The array of doctors your Attending Physician refers you to might help you regain some cognitive functioning, and set you on the right medical course for recovery. At the same time, your Case Manager should refer you, as necessary, to the appropriate therapists and lawyers, which is the subject of the next chapter.

15 – Building Your Recovery Team: REHABILITATION

OVERVIEW

A good Case Manager should be able to refer you to the right therapists and even neurolawyers as necessary.

Figure 7:

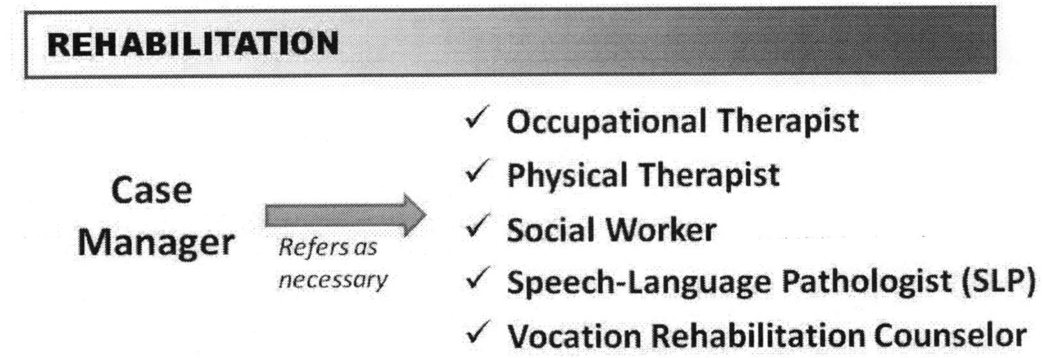

OCCUPATIONAL THERAPIST

Occupational Therapists (OT) often get confused with Vocational Therapists because they both sound job-related. Although "occupational" in this context can mean vocational or job-related, it more frequently refers to any meaningful activity that people do, including taking care of oneself, running errands, engaging in leisure activities, driving and participating in educational experiences.

Activities of Daily Living (ADLs)

OTs help TBI patients determine their ability to perform what are called ADLs – Activities of Daily Living – and then work together to find ways of performing them. The extent of the OT's involvement depends on the severity of the injury. Because mild TBI survivors usually have little problem with such ADLs as brushing teeth, getting dressed and bathing, OTs most often are part of the recovery team for moderate to severe cases of TBI.

Although some TBI patients are never referred to an Occupational Therapist (OT), many activities can be made much easier with an OT's help. For example, survivors often find grocery shopping overwhelming because of the noise, bright lights, scanning of labels and decision-making. OTs see this as an intervention opportunity: it is both a means to an end – an opportunity to practice cognitive strategies – as well as an end in itself because people need to be able to go grocery shopping. OTs help develop strategies specific to the survivor for getting in and out of a grocery store with a minimum of overstimulation and cognitive strain.

Physical, cognitive and/or psychosocial challenges

OTs work with a wide range of TBI survivors who have physical, cognitive and/or psychosocial challenges.

OTs help TBI survivors with physical challenges:

- Move their arms and hands, sometimes making splints for them if necessary;

- With balance problems, figure out how to get around their home environment; for example, working in the kitchen, and getting in and out of the tub and car;

- Compensate for residual physical problems, such as figuring out how to get dressed again, drive again, take care of the household again, and so on.

OTs help TBI survivors with cognitive challenges:

- Organize and sequence daily living tasks in order to simplify and compensate for thinking challenges;

- Use compensatory strategies for short-term memory problems during daily activities.

OTs help TBI survivors with psychosocial challenges:

- Deal with PTSD related to TBI as it shows up in daily activities;

- Cope with life changes related to TBI, including relationship stressors.

Cranial sacral therapy

Gregg was quite enthusiastic about an OT he began seeing at Spaulding. She told him – and this at first struck both of us as a bit extreme – that every half hour he should stop what he's doing, evaluate how he's feeling, and if he feels at all as though he's straining, he should meditate for 10 or 15 minutes. He started doing this and he found it to be a very useful plan. I tried something close to this, and after using this kind of strategy for awhile, you begin to internalize it, and learn to pace yourself through every strenuous activity.

His OT also performed wonders in the area of cranial sacral therapy. I thought I should try this and so I made a few appointments with her colleague. She would have me lay down on a cot in a small cordoned-off area in a large room, and then she would place her hands under me. Beginning at my feet, she would work her way up to the top of my head; under my legs, under my lower back and then upper back, under my shoulders and neck, and then under the heaviest part of my skull.

From foot to head this took about 20 minutes. Then she would leave me alone for the rest of the hour and I would be in a deep, blissful state. I could hear things happening in the room but it all sounded far, far away. It's the only time when I have started dreaming and not been asleep. It could only have been a healing experience.

Return-to-work preparation

Occupational Therapists also use what's called "assistive technology" to train survivors on how to begin to re-engage in the activities they value the most. A good example of that would be voice-recognition software to eliminate the need to type. OTs have the long view of preparing survivors for returning to work, and at some point a Vocational Therapist might move to the forefront of the recovery team.

For more on the OT's role in recovery, go to The American Occupational Therapy Association, Inc.'s site at www.aota.org.

PHYSICAL THERAPIST

The more severe the brain injury, the likelier it is that the survivor's body is affected. As with other therapists on this list, some TBI patients are never referred to a Physical Therapist (PT) even though a PT trained in brain-injury rehabilitation can be a huge help in improving the quality of life. As the name suggests, a PT gets involved with all aspects of overcoming a survivor's physical challenges.

These sessions might include improving balance, increasing upper- and lower-body strength, and achieving better endurance, all of which can help the survivor live more independently. PTs can come to your home if mobility is a problem, and look into providing special equipment you might need for a home-exercise regimen.

For more on the PT's role in recovery, go to the American Physical Therapy Association's site at www.apta.org.

SOCIAL WORKER

Your Social Worker helps you address your social concerns, but since "social" is pretty abstract; let's talk particulars.

Family

She can advise you about how to improve your relationship with your spouse or partner; for example, "My husband is upset about how my injury has shrunk our social life. How do we cope?" She will work directly with your partner and meet with you either as a couple or individually.

The first time Lynne came with me to meet Sally Johnson, my social worker, Sally directed most of the questions to her. Lynne told me later that she was glad Sally hadn't tried to establish too much intimacy right away. After all, this *is* New England!

Sally also included our boys in the discussion, asking questions about how they were coping with the changes that have taken place in our family as a result of my injury. On the way home Lynne said that it was good to have a time and place to talk about family issues because we might not have raised them otherwise.

Months later, when I asked Lynne if she could go with me again to see Sally – I had been seeing her every three weeks alone – she said, "Why, so I can hear about all the things I'm doing wrong?" She meant it to be funny, but the underlying truth was that because Sally and I had established a good working relationship, Lynne did feel a little like an outsider. You will want to consider that dynamic, and make sure your partner does not feel threatened or alienated. If this is the case, consider where your partner can get support.

Friends

You might be worried about losing your friends because it's so hard for you to interact socially. Your social worker will help you retain friendships by suggesting coping tactics and ideas about what to say in various situations. Sally helped me figure out what behaviors were helpful. For example, at our house I can retire early and our friends understand. "Goodnight, everyone!" "Goodnight John!" You will want to take notes on your visits to your social worker so you can remember all her tips.

Work

Your social worker can help you address your concerns about missing work or underperforming at work. They can help you answer questions such as: What do I tell my boss about why I can't make the deadline? My colleagues say things that make me think they believe I'm a slacker. How do I respond?

They will also be on the alert for any signs of depression, and might recommend evaluation for possible medical intervention. This is a big advantage of being treated in a rehabilitation hospital like Spaulding in Boston. All or most of your recovery team share your file, and communicate with each other on your behalf.

SPEECH-LANGUAGE PATHOLOGIST (SLP)

"Speech-language pathology" might actually be a bit misleading because your SLP might do a lot more than help you with speech problems such as stuttering and stammering. If he's good, and mine was very good, your SLP can address all the areas where you struggle cognitively, such as how you problem-solve and reason, how you process and retain information, and how you communicate it, whether reading it, writing it, or speaking it.

This might seem pretty abstract, but in practical terms it means that your SLP is the knight who rides up on the white horse to rescue you:

- If your short-term memory seems to have evaporated;

- If you're unable to sustain a conversation even with a close family member;

- If you find it impossible to read your favorite mysteries anymore;

- If it's hard for you to concentrate – specially in emotionally charged or socially demanding situations where you're also under time pressure;

- If your efforts to do any of these things totally exhaust you.

SLP testing, and the price you pay

Make an appointment with a reputable SLP as soon as you are diagnosed with mild TBI. They will perform a battery of tests to identify your brain strengths and deficiencies. Just as neuropsych tests help to quantify aspects of this "invisible injury," so too will your work with your SLP. Be prepared: Some of the SLP's findings might upset you.

One of my lowest days came after I scored high on some reading comprehension tests – 99th percentile, the best that Rick Sanders, my SLP, had ever seen. My high score depressed me because it was like when you were a little kid and you felt miserable, but your temperature is a solid 98.6 degrees. You desperately want the SLP tests to prove you're injured, so when a test comes up with nothing, you tend to feel isolated and might even find yourself wondering yet again, *am I crazy?*

Rick had this to say:

> I probably made (or I customarily make) a comment that the tests give us a window into a certain kind of performance, but that the tests don't mirror real life. They are short, you're usually given the directions, and as you have said, John, they don't measure any after effects.
>
> So we can't use them as the final word – just one piece of information to help our understanding. So I certainly believe someone – and try to communicate this – when they tell me they have problems doing work

> or home-related tasks, even if their test scores are good. I hope I tried
> to help you not to feel bad about these tests.

A high score on an SLP or neuropsych test says nothing about the cognitive strain and fatigue you have to struggle with while you're taking them and the crash you might experience afterwards. Before testing, tell your family that you will need quiet and solitude for several hours and perhaps days after testing to facilitate your recovery.

Stay the course because many tests provide snapshots of different aspects of cognitive functioning. These include tests such as math, verbal and reading comprehension assessments; reading summaries both written and oral; and logic puzzles. I also took tests of concentration and complex attention, memory and speed of processing information. These kinds of tests can, with startling precision, identify the parts of the brain that the injury affected.

SLP testing quantifies changes in your brain over time

For example, your SLP might ask you to do a logic puzzle. She'll observe and time you, and when you complete it she'll note the date and the length of time it took you. Three months later, and then six months later, she might ask you to repeat the test. Compiling the results over time allows her to identify improvements, declines, or deficiencies.

Your SLP tests you so she can identify the tactics and strategies that can help you address your deficiencies. During one very early session Rick was telling me something so useful that I reached into my pocket for a scrap of paper so I could write it down. When I started to write on it he asked me, "Where's your notebook?" I told him I'd left it at home since we were just doing testing. Rick said, "Your notebook is a prosthesis for your brain. You'll find it helpful to always carry it with you. It will make a lot of things easier for you."

Rick turned out to be right. I have carried my notebook with me ever since and on multiple levels it has made my life a lot easier. Over and over, your SLP will say something like this: "Okay, we've figured out that you have trouble doing this task. Here's what you can do to make it easier…." In fact, the key strategy from your SLP is, "Make it easy on your brain."

VOCATIONAL REHABILITATION COUNSELOR

If you're planning to return to the job you were doing before your injury or if you're anxious about being able to function on your old job, you should have a vocational rehab counselor on your team. A vocational rehab counselor is trained to help you make informed decisions every step of the way as you consider your employment future and think about your vocational goals.

As Seattle-based Dr. Robert Fraser explains, these specialists can help you ask yourself the big questions, such as, "Can I actually function on my old job or should I think about a new job? What kinds of training and support are available to me in either case?" As I said earlier, be sure he or she has training in and experience working with TBI patients.

Your vocational rehab counselor has an impressive toolkit

Your counselor can help you answer lots of additional questions using the wide variety of tools in her vocational rehab toolkit. For example, if you haven't had neuropsychological testing, they can arrange that for you. They can work directly with you, your other team members, and even with potential employers to help you think clearly about your job opportunities in relation to your cognitive and physical strengths and weaknesses.

Through their array of resources they can help you find work that's right for you, and even assist you with challenges such as transportation. They can explain the support options available to you once you take on a job, such as one-on-one job coaching, work station and schedule changes to accommodate your disabilities, and sophisticated software technologies that can help to compensate for your deficits.

A vocational rehabilitation counselor also brings her extensive knowledge of disability and employment law to your particular situation. She knows all about Social Security and other federal disability laws, as well as the laws associated with employment in your state and how they will apply to you. Did you know, for example, that one Department of Labor law allows you to "test drive" different jobs for a specified time period on an unpaid basis to see if they fit you? Best of all, the state fully pays for many of the services this person offers.

Contact her

Do an online search for "vocational rehabilitation counselor" and the name of your state and you'll come up with the website you need to contact a counselor. Do you live in the city? Make an appointment with a vocational rehab counselor in the office nearest you. Do you live in the country? A vocational rehab counselor will come to you[29].

A RECOVERY TEAM MEMBER CAN SERVE AS YOUR CASE MANAGER

Any member of your recovery team can function informally as your Case Manager, although there is formal certification in "case management." You might decide you want to have your social worker be your Case Manager. Your Case Manager is your "go-to" person. She helps you to plan, coordinate and evaluate the ongoing services of your medical team so that you get the best of care in the most cost-effective fashion.

Recovering from a brain injury is a full-time job, and your Case Manager can serve as a much-needed assistant. In fact, you can think of your Case Manager as the hub of your recovery team. For example, she'll guide you in these ways:

- "You need to see Dr. D to deal with your sleep issue."

- "I'll set up an appointment for you with Dr. G to help you deal with depression."

- "You mentioned the problem you are having with the computer screen – Dr. Z is very good with vision problems."

As I've said, my neurotrauma rehab specialist, Beth Adams, serves as my Case Manager. In one instance she actually walked me down the hall of the rehab hospital where I was being treated to see if I could meet with a particular doctor about an emerging problem. The next time I met with her she asked for the details of that meeting, and when she felt it was important to have three members of the team talk openly with each other, she arranged and led a conference call with them.

Acting as my quarterback in the first several years of my recovery, she had me come back to the huddle about once a month to update her about the latest developments in my life.

NEUROLAWYER (BRAIN INJURY LAWYER)

TBI survivors often face lifelong financial challenges. These include lost income and medical/rehabilitation costs, and legal obstacles to obtaining disability insurance, unemployment benefits and personal injury awards. My attorney, Kenneth L. Kolpan, told me:

> Persons who incur head injury will necessarily face legal problems as a result of their injury. The nature of the injury with its resultant treatment, as well as the cause of the injury (often a motor vehicle accident), leads to involvement in the legal system . . . A person's ability to access medical treatment, insurance coverage and personal injury compensation is affected by the law.

It is essential to have a lawyer who specializes in brain injury litigation – or neurolaw, as it is sometimes called – on your recovery team. He or she will use experts on brain injury such as neuropsychologists, neuropsychiatrists, physiatrists (doctors who draw on multiple disciplines to help people recover from lost functioning due to illness or injury), and speech-language pathologists to "advocate for you" so you receive "just compensation" for a brain injury caused by injury.

Kolpan also said:

> Brain injury cases are unique, challenging and complex. It is essential to have well experienced legal representation by an attorney who concentrates his practice in brain injury litigation…

> The attorney must be familiar with the mechanism of how brain injuries occur… have access to brain injury experts who can teach jurors, judges and adjusters about the consequences of brain injuries…and the background to handle these complex, challenging and sometimes difficult cases.

Contact the Brain Injury Association in your state and/or ask local providers in the brain injury rehabilitation community for a recommendation. Word of mouth from other TBI survivors can also be a good route.

Make sure the lawyer has experience representing survivors of brain injury

The first lawyer I contacted was a friend of mine who said that he could help me sort out all the legal issues. Lynne, however, wisely considered the possible fallout to the friendship if the legal aspect ended badly. I e-mailed him and explained the awkwardness – a cognitive effort that laid me out the rest of the day – and asked if he could recommend someone. Lynne and I drove to Worcester and met with his friend, a high-powered attorney who had represented clients before the State Supreme Court.

We spent an hour and a half with him, tearfully telling him everything about the accident and the horrible fallout of Andrew's and my injuries. After listening to all of this, he said, "You know, if this ever went to trial, it would help if you were at least wearing a neck brace or something because you look fine."

If your lawyer says this, consider it a red flag. It means he does not understand that TBI is an "invisible injury."

The kind of neurolawyer you want

Lynne and I talked the whole ride home about how unsettling his final comment was. She said we should ask my Case Manager if she knew anyone familiar with brain injury, specifically mild brain injury. She promptly put me in touch with Kolpan in Boston, who used to teach at Tufts Medical School. He would never suggest a neck brace for the sake of the jury because he knows how to explain TBI – mild or otherwise – in clear, specific terms.

Kolpan is a widely known and respected brain injury lawyer who has been advocating for the rights of TBI survivors for almost three decades and was recently elected president of the Massachusetts Brain Injury Association.[30] He truly understands the world of mild TBI in all its daunting complexity. I encouraged a fellow TBI'er to spend time on Kolpan's website, and his response was, "Man, he gets it! He really gets it!"

A brain injury attorney understands that mild TBI'ers can undermine their own legal cases because they look normal. As Kolpan observed, "The person with TBI might be his or her own worst witness." Your neurolawyer will prove to a judge and jury that although your "mild" (or "minor") TBI might be invisible due to a "clean" CT scan, EEG, X-ray, or PET scan, it is real nonetheless, and devastating.

If your neurolawyer does win a settlement, your financial pressures will ease and you can direct your limited energy and attention to your recovery. (Note: Although I did not press criminal charges, and there was no settlement for us to win, Kolpan expertly guided us through the arcane and arduous process of communicating with the insurance company of the guy who hit us.)

The nearest city might be a better place to look than locally

Arthur, Tom's partner from Chapter 2, makes this point:

> Identify lawyers and medical providers who recognize and have expertise with this kind of injury so you don't have to convince them of its reality.
>
> You know how many hours I had to try to explain – and argue about – Tom's condition to lawyers? We made the mistake of looking locally for attorneys. We didn't realize that the best lawyers who understand post- accident effects on the brain in our state are in the Boston area, and that they travel to research and argue their cases.
>
> Knowing what we know now, we should have sought out the best attorneys in Boston instead of in the small city close to us. Every local lawyer we met with knew nothing about Tom's post-injury problems.

Specialties within neurolaw

I asked Kolpan about two legal issues: applying for Social Security Disability Benefits, and reading my employer's statement of long-term disability benefits. He referred me to two separate neurolawyers to handle these areas for me. It speaks well of Kolpan, too, that he didn't wing it and say he'd take care of them both for me.

One attorney came with me to my Social Security hearing, and he ended up not saying a word. Apparently, my case was black and white. The other attorney worked with me to determine what I could expect from my employer during the first two years of my injury.

It might not be too late for you to contact a neurolawyer

Even if it took you years to be diagnosed with TBI, it's worth contacting a neurolawyer. Kolpan told me:

> The Statute of Limitations defines the time limit during which a head-injured person can file a lawsuit.
>
> The Statute has two main purposes: to make sure that any potential defendants are not forever at risk for a lawsuit and to encourage that legitimate lawsuits be filed while memories and evidence are fresh.
>
> Depending on the type of lawsuit, the Statute of Limitations can be any number of years. Once the time limit has passed, no suit can be started.
>
> The time period at which the Statute of Limitations begins to run is crucial. Does it begin when the person is injured or when the person discovers he or she is injured? State laws vary.
>
> Once the time limit begins, some laws lift the time limit while the injured person is disabled or incompetent and then resume the time period when the disability is removed.
>
> However, some states mandate an outer limit of time even when a disability tolls the time limit (known as a Statute of Repose).

A neurolawyer will tell you about the Statute of Limitations in your state.

16 – Making the Most of Your Appointments

HAVE A CAREGIVER JOIN YOU

Your Attending Physician and Case Manager want to help you – in fact they're in the business of helping you – but it's up to you to provide specific information about your injury, and your day-to-day life since the day of your incident. But your brain injury probably makes it hard for you to communicate clearly, so consider having a caregiver, advocate, or support person accompany you to your appointments with your Attending Physician and Case Manager. I noticed a distinct improvement in the quality of my interactions and meetings after Lynne started going with me.

To ensure that clear and accurate information is being communicated in both directions in your appointments, your designated caregiver can:

- Set up a tape recorder, if you both think that could be useful;

- Take notes so that you can focus on your interaction;

- Help to ensure that you are treated fairly and with respect.

Rick Sanders agrees:

> This is invaluable advice. I worked with a man who was hit by a drunk driver, with broken bones in the clavicle and shoulder. The MD would ask him how his shoulder was – and if he had no pain at that time the man would say that it was fine. [His wife] would then remind him that he was up all night in pain. She was then looked at as if she were the hysterical wife, since the patient said he was fine.

Although the doctor might have initially have assumed some kind of hysteria on her part, it was essential that he hear from both patient and spouse about the reality of the injury.

Rick also makes these recommendations:

- If you use a daily planner, bring it with you to doctor appointments.

- Make preparatory notes and questions you want to address with your doctor.

- Open the planner during the visit and refer to these notes.

- Jot down important points.

- If it is hard for you to listen, think and make notes at the same time, tell your doctor that this is the case and ask him to write down the answers to your questions in your planner.

- If the doctor is reluctant to take that time, then ask for a copy of the note he will write about that visit, including the relevant responses to your questions.

CHECKLIST: MAKING THE MOST OF YOUR APPOINTMENTS

This checklist will help you make the most of your appointments with your Attending Physician and Case Manager. You might want to bring these pages with you and refer to them during your appointments. Consider copying them and giving them to your Attending Physician and Case Manager so they know how they can help you make the most of your meetings.

Expect your Attending Physician and Case Manager to partner with you by providing a reasonable level of emotional support, informed guidance and tactical support. Each bullet point is described on the pages that follow.

Emotional Support	<ul><li>Anticipate how you're feeling and respond with empathy.</li><li>Assure you that what you're experiencing is normal – normal for someone with a brain injury.</li><li>Give you pep talks.</li><li>Support your decision to bring a relative or friend to your appointments.</li></ul>
Informed Guidance	<ul><li>Learn about your injury from you.</li><li>Be humble and utterly professional.</li><li>Stick to their profession.</li><li>Help you watch for signs of clinical depression and thoughts of suicide.</li></ul>
Tactical Support	<ul><li>Refer you to specialists as part of your recovery team.</li><li>Identify the tests that will help evaluate and treat your sequelae.</li><li>Provide a note to your employer about your absence.</li><li>Help you see that some cognitive exertions might be worth the aftermath.</li><li>Encourage you to improve your physical fitness.</li><li>Identify ways for you to pace yourself throughout the day.</li><li>Help you consider carefully whether to try prescribed medications.</li></ul>

EMOTIONAL SUPPORT

Expect your Attending Physician and Case Manager to partner with you by providing a reasonable level of <u>emotional support</u>.

Guideline	Explanation
Anticipate how you're feeling and respond with empathy	• Your advocate should say to you, "Tell the doctor specifically how your injury is affecting you." • Have your advocate watch for condescending, dismissive, or skeptical tones in their voice. • If necessary, your advocate can ask them to use a positive, supportive and encouraging tone; and to make eye contact to connect with you and to show they are listening.
Assure you that what you're experiencing is normal . . . normal for someone with a brain injury	• Ask for their advice about how to cope with the loneliness that TBI patients experience. • Ask them how to balance your need for quiet and isolation with your need for interaction.
Give you pep talks	• Tell them that you always benefit from encouragement. • Tell them that you are easily discouraged.
Support your decision to bring a relative or friend to your appointments	• Tell them that your advocate will be the designated note-taker and, if necessary, speak for you when your TBI makes communication hard.

Other things I need:

INFORMED GUIDANCE

Expect your Attending Physician and Case Manager to partner with you by providing a reasonable level of <u>informed guidance</u>.

Guideline	Explanation
Learn about your injury from you	• If they greet you with "You look great!" remind them that mild TBI is invisible, and that you don't feel great. • Remind them that every brain injury is different, leaving a unique "fingerprint." • Ask them to note the sequelae you describe that might be unique to you. • Ask them to draw on their experience treating others with similar sequelae. • Ask that they seek information about your injury from you, and not only from academic journals.
Stick to their profession	• They should address only the problems that are within their professional expertise. • They should ask "checklist"-type questions to determine whether you need other professional help; e.g.: "Are you feeling depressed?" If you answer "Yes, I'm depressed," they should refer you to an expert.
Help you watch for signs of clinical depression and thoughts of suicide	• Tell them immediately if you are depressed or have any suicidal thoughts. • As appropriate, have your advocate share observations and concerns, and ask questions. • Work with your advocate and doctor to decide whether you should see a neuropsychiatrist.

INFORMED GUIDANCE *(CONT'D)*

Guideline	Explanation
Be humble and utterly professional	• Tell them that their receptivity to what you say assures you that you are in good hands. • If other doctors have attributed your sequelae to something other than a brain injury, say so. Be specific. • If their attentiveness distinguishes them from others you've seen, thank them. • Request that they make the best use of your time by helping you stay focused. • Keep in mind: the best professionals display curiosity and ask you a lot of questions. • They should never respond dismissively to any issue that you bring up – each is important. Even say something as simple as, "Please hear what I'm saying." • If they say, "You should be well by now," remind them that many survivors have long-term sequelae.

Other things I need:

TACTICAL SUPPORT

Expect your Attending Physician and Case Manager to partner with you by providing a reasonable level of <u>tactical support</u>.

Guideline	Explanation
Refer you to specialists as part of your recovery team	• Ask yourself whether you feel that you are in good hands. If you don't, have your advocate help you ask your Attending Physician and Case Manager how to restore your confidence in your recovery. • Ask your Attending Physician to refer you for a sleep study and vestibular testing, and to explain how these specialists can contribute to your diagnosis and recovery: Endocrinologist, Neuropsychiatrist, Neuropsychologist and Psychopharmacologist. • Ask your Case Manager to explain how these specialists can contribute to your recovery and rehabilitation: NeuroLawyer, Social Worker, Speech-Language Pathologist (SLP) and Vocational Rehabilitation Counselor.
Identify the tests that will help evaluate and treat your sequelae	• At a minimum, at the first sign of concussion or brain injury, you should undergo a CT scan, MRI and EEG. Even if these tests show no brain damage, it provides a starting point for diagnosis. • Understand this: It is great news if these tests do not show damage to the brain, but it does not mean you do not have a traumatic brain injury.
Provide a note to your employer about your absence	• For example: "Joe's recovery team has not cleared him to return to work yet." • A note helps reduce your stress about your inability to work, relieves you of having to explain your absence yourself, and legitimizes your "invisible injury" to colleagues.

TACTICAL SUPPORT *(CONT'D)*

Guideline	Explanation
Help you see that some cognitive exertions might be worth the aftermath	• Ask them to advise you on how to approach interactions such as having dinner with friends, running errands for your family, attending support-group meetings, or attending a child's school event. • Ask for advice on how to cope with any resulting fallout from cognitive exertion.
Encourage you to improve your physical fitness	• Ask them to explain the benefits of improving your physical fitness, including improved blood flow, brain health, and feeling and looking better. • Ask them for ideas on the best approach given your limitations: e.g., balance problems or fatigue.
Identify ways for you to pace yourself throughout the day	• Ask for advice on how to resume former activities, and how you can gauge when you're doing too much. • Ask for advice on how to cope with the "crash" if you do too much.
Help you consider carefully whether to try prescribed medications	• Have them explain how a stimulant such as Ritalin might benefit you without overly agitating your injured brain. • Have them explain how an antidepressant might benefit you. • Make sure that every member of your recovery team knows what medications you are on.

Other things I need:

17 – Highlights of Strategy Sessions

OVERVIEW

Because most survivors do not have the opportunity to work with some of the best professionals in the field, I thought of calling this chapter "Spaulding in a Box." It highlights the many strategy sessions I've had with my D.O., Case Manager, SLP and Social Worker.

Because this chapter is over a dozen pages long, here are the six most important highlights upfront:

1. Pace yourself

Remember the nature of your injury. Your brain is not like a bicep that gets stronger when you work it until it hurts. Think of your brain more like an injury to your Achilles tendon. You make it worse when you cause it pain. Pain is your brain's way of saying, "Stop!"

The harder lesson to learn, especially for high-achieving people, is to stop *before* your brain hurts. Pay attention to the clock, and figure out how many minutes to give yourself before you stop what you are doing, even if 1) you are not finished and 2) your brain does not hurt yet.

Most hikers live by the rule, "Drink before you feel thirsty" because dehydration has already begun to set in by the time your body registers thirst. Plan your rest times in advance. Schedule them the way you would any other important event. Make a draining activity like bill-paying or filing *time-based*, not based on whether you've completed it.

2. Count the cost of every activity

Measure your time like money. Every task you perform exacts a cost from you. Calculate whether what you plan to do will be worth the inevitable crash.

3. Don't be hard on yourself

Make your goals modest and achievable. Encourage your caregiver to help you look for "wins"; something you did that was positive, and that might be a sign of progress in your recovery. Remember that depression lurks behind every corner and you must recognize signs of it and fight it. Your mental health is a fabric that can be unraveled very quickly if you pick at a single thread.

For example, stop yourself when you hear your mind's voice say something like, "Well that was stupid!" You've got enough going on in your life right now, and you are trying so very hard that the last thing you need is to be insulting yourself. You are not crazy, you are not lazy, and you are not stupid. You have a brain injury.

4. Write things down

Don't rely on your memory anymore. It has probably become unreliable. Record important events and commitments on a calendar or journal, and bring it with you wherever you go. This will relieve you of the emotional stress and cognitive strain of trying to remember something. Once you've written it down, your mind is free to simply think again, and not be burdened with anxiety.

5. Avoid isolation

It is easier for many survivors to be alone than to interact with people, but loneliness is one of the most crushing aspects of a brain injury. Make sure you seek out connections with people you find relatively easy to be with. Keep in mind the environment in which you will meet, and make sure it is not noisy or oppressively lit. Some survivors have found that online social networking such as Facebook helps reduce these feelings of isolation because communications are on their own controlled terms.

6. Be hopeful

Remember that most people do recover from a brain injury. If you are in the minority who do not recover – and even this minority number is huge – many resources and supports are available for you. Start by searching for brain-injury resources in your state, and contact your state's Brain Injury Association and/or the Brain Injury Association of America.

SESSIONS WITH MY D.O.

I am extremely fortunate that my D.O. (Doctor of Osteopathy) is Ross Zafonte, a prominent brain-injury specialist at Spaulding Rehabilitation Hospital. He has published extensively on TBIs, spasticity, and other neurological disorders.[31] In addition to his duties at Spaulding – Vice President of Research and Education – he also serves as Chair of the Department of Physical Medicine and Rehabilitation (PMR) at Harvard Medical School. I meet with him every three months and we fine-tune my treatment.

A few key points

In March 2011, Dr Zafonte was the keynote speaker at the Massachusetts BIA's annual conference. Much of it covered some pretty technical TBI research findings but he made some memorable points for those of us able to follow along:

- A brain injury occurs once every 16 seconds in North America.

- That is the equivalent of all of the passengers of five 747's suffering a brain injury every day.

- Traumatic brain injury is not an event; it's a disease. It is a process, not an event.

- During a course of treatment, consider carefully, realistically and in a timely way whether or not it is working for you. The intention is always to "target the right person at the right time."

Alcohol as neurotoxin

Dr Zafonte has pointed out what now seem like some pretty basic steps to facilitate healing of my brain, including vigorous exercise and good nutrition. At one early meeting, I told him about a particularly odious stretch, and said it was after a very quiet evening with friends. I had enjoyed a glass of wine and conversation, but nothing more stimulating than that.

It was then that he told me to avoid alcohol, which he calls a neurotoxin for TBI survivors. This was the first time I'd heard this, and I was five years into my recovery. When your brain is making your life miserable, even the word "neurotoxin" *sounds* painful. He explained that alcohol harms brain tissue in several ways and can interfere with medications. (For more on this, see my website www.tbistrategies.com.)

Resting when it feels premature to rest

I come to our sessions prepared to tell him highlights – which are mostly lowlights – of the past 3 months, and we discuss the possible causes and ramifications. For example, I tell him about periods of over-exertion, when very early the next day I experience a "lead blanket" drape over me and I have to lie down on and off all day. These exert/crash cycles are intense, and we talk about how to mitigate them. After a sidebar conversation about cholesterol, in which I told him about lowering mine from 275 to 150 without medication – using only natural remedies – he said, "Rest is as prophylactic as cayenne pepper." I think that was the first time I had heard "prophylactic" used that way.

He emphasizes, as do Rick Sanders and Sally Johnson, the need to rest *before* feeling terrible. This is a simple strategy, but one that survivors often ignore, myself included. We are hard-wired to rest only when we're tired. This is why it's smart to refer to a clock, and time your exertions rather than think, "I'll stop when the job is done, or when I feel I need to."

Dr. Zafonte also agrees that survivors who are used to being – and miss being – high-performers have an especially difficult time in their recovery. When the neurosurgeon told me a week after my accident to "go home and do nothing for three weeks," what did that mean exactly? At the time, it meant shutting out as much visual and auditory stimulation as possible to allow the brain to focus itself on healing. But how should we live our lives now, some number of years into our recovery? These stimulations are still harsh for us, and many of us get frustrated at our inability to function at a high level on any given day. Anything we do seems to exact a price.

One answer is to rest before we feel the need to. This takes an odd kind of discipline. It's different, obviously, than the discipline we normally use to push ourselves to ordinary or extraordinary heights of accomplishment. This is common training for life, and one we have to somehow unlearn if we are serious about facilitating healing and recovery. Although initially it felt very much like defeat for me, there should be no shame for the survivor to say at various points in the day, "I'm going to go rest now." It should be a point of pride that you are practicing the discipline of rest.

Light-emitting diode therapy (LED)

I have participated in certain aspects of Dr Zafonte's research, and I try the new, and in some instances experimental, therapies he suggests. For instance, he asked whether I would be willing to try LED therapy three days a week for six weeks. I jumped at the chance for some kind of improvement, both in terms of cognition and mood.

The first two weeks were brutal, weeks three and four brought possible improvements, but then during weeks five and six I felt as though the lights were burning my brain, actually singeing it in some way. That was probably my imagination but that is how it felt. Although we agreed that LED therapy was not measurably helping me, it might help other TBI survivors.

Anticipatory theory

A hockey fan, Dr. Zafonte told me about what he calls "anticipatory theory," citing Wayne "the Great One" Gretsky's endless sessions of attacking the puck with his stick as it flew off the walls of the ice and swooping it into the net. Gretsky became so adept at reading the puck's flight by learning to anticipate where the puck would be after hitting it into the wall at an almost infinite number of angles and speed. So, too, in our recovery, we must learn to anticipate how a certain activity, whether we consider it work or pleasure, will affect our next few hours or days.

SESSIONS WITH MY CASE MANAGER

As I've said, Beth Adams has been my Case Manager from the beginning. Beth is a nationally recognized Neurotrauma Rehabilitation Specialist in the Boston area and Salem MA who provides specialized and individualized rehabilitation services to those who have sustained a concussion or traumatic brain injury. She is on the Medical Advisory Committee for the Retired Boxers Foundation, and is the Neurocognitive Assessment Specialist at the Brigham and Women Neurological Sports Injury Center.

I started seeing her shortly after the neurosurgeon referred me to her. Lynne came with me. One great thing about seeing Beth once a month was that she noted progress each time she saw me. She called them "bigger than baby steps." You and even your family might not see improvements, but your Case Manager will have a whole month's worth of improvements to tell you about and encourage you with.

She also helped me put a positive spin on certain observations I would make about my own sense of progress. For example, I told her I'd become frustrated when I tried to do some simple math in my head and that I'd resorted to using a calculator. She smiled brightly and told me that I had problem-solved. I hadn't just frozen and sat there defeated. I actively sought out a solution. She encouraged me with that insight because I was also noticing that problem-solving was not my strong suit anymore.

She gave me some important things to keep in mind, including:

- Neurologists focus on the acute event, and don't always see the whole rehab process. Don't worry about that because you'll have other rehab professionals on your team.

- Occasionally ask to see copies of your medical records. Sometimes doctors word things vaguely and can be misinterpreted, say by insurance reps or other members of your recovery team. For example, "John is writing a book" can imply that you are not suffering every day with a brain injury. You need to clarify, if necessary, your extremely small windows of productivity and the aftermath of what writing does to you.

- When someone asks, "When are you going back to work?" simply say, "I haven't been given the okay to return to work," or "My recovery team has not approved my return to work yet." Don't put the burden on your shoulders in addition to everything else you are going through. Not working is not a choice you are making.

- Begin the process of Social Security Disability. You have to have been disabled for at least a year, and early on you won't know how long you will suffer with the injury, so get the process started. A survivor might be denied two or three times via the mail, and then you have the option to appear before a judge.

- Social Security allows for a person who receives disability income to engage in "trial work," which it considers practice for real work while continuing to receive Social Security Disability Income (SSDI).

- In the world of vocational rehabilitation, you hear words like "functional abilities" and "functional limitations". Your first projects when you return to work should play to your strengths.

- You might run across the term "MME". It stands for Maximum Medical Endpoint, which is the medical profession's way of saying, "We've done all we can."

- Legally, employers who take back employees after disability leave must provide "reasonable accommodation" to their injury that will allow them to perform essential job functions.*

- The term "community model" refers to incorporating skills learned during rehabilitation into day-to-day life. A survivor's goal is not to be a great patient but to transfer skills into community life.

- If you don't use the strategies you are learning, you buck the system you need.

* According to the U.S. Department of Justice:

> A reasonable accommodation is any modification or adjustment to a job or the work environment that will enable a qualified applicant or employee with a disability to participate in the application process or to perform essential job functions.
>
> Reasonable accommodation also includes adjustments to assure that a qualified individual with a disability has rights and privileges in employment equal to those of employees without disabilities.

SESSIONS WITH MY SPEECH-LANGUAGE PATHOLOGIST (SLP)[32]

"We would never expect someone with a broken leg to run a marathon."

Rick Sanders

Rick has been my right-hand man throughout this recovery and rehab. He's been working with people like me – and people a lot worse off than me – for over 25 years. In addition to his Master's Degree in SLP, he also has one in Theological Studies from Harvard Divinity School across the Charles River in Cambridge. As you can imagine, our conversations can get pretty wide-ranging. He's the salt of the earth. After I spoke to a roomful of Case Managers, a woman came up to me and said her son had been in a terrible car accident, and after seeing a number of specialists, Rick was the only one who taught him to speak again.

Once, after Rick and I had worked together a few times, I walked into his office and he stood there smiling at me. He looked me right in the eye and asked, "How are you?" I groaned because I knew that he knew that was the question I had problems answering. He kept smiling and asked, rather perversely I thought, "Well . . . how are you?"

I tried to answer as best I could, like a kid learning how to swim in the deep end. What Rick made clear to me was that his office would be a low-risk environment to try things. In our sessions he sometimes puts me on the spot, the same spot as in real life, and has me practice what I would say when somebody asks me that kind of open-ended question.

Rick has become part cognitive therapist and part personal trainer, as though he's pushing me to do more pull-ups or run another lap. However, Rick doesn't push my fragile brain to the point of damaging me; he has helped me understand the consequences of pushing myself.

Metaphors

Using metaphors to describe what is hard to describe really helps, and Rick taught me some great ones.

- He calls that place in our brains that stores short-term memories our mental clipboard. Say you're adding 12 + 32 and then have to add 9 to it. You have to hold onto 44 before you can add the 9. You have to put 44 onto your clipboard. Well, brain-injured people have smaller clipboards now; we can't hold onto and retrieve information as easily as we could before the injury, even something as simple as a series of numbers or four random words.

- Rick compares memory to Velcro because brain injuries can make our memories slippery, with no little hooks for them to latch onto.

- When I told Rick about one especially busy day I'd had, which was followed by some very bad days in a row, he said, "We would never expect someone with a broken leg to run a marathon."

"Flooding"

Rick attached new words to my experiences and feelings, and this gave them validity. If there was a word for an experience or a feeling, it meant that my feelings and experiences weren't unique to me, and therefore, I wasn't "crazy." Other people were having the same experiences and feelings.

"Flooding" was that kind of word, and a useful metaphor. When I would bump up against something beyond me, like instructions or trying to explain something, my mind would feel jammed and because I was watching that happen to me, I tended to get all choked up about it. "How sad!" I would think, and then that line from Pink Floyd again, "This is not who I am." I wouldn't be able to go any further.

For example, try taking a minute to call out as many words as you can beginning with the letter "a." You probably came up with a lot more than four, which is all I could manage early on. As a professional writer, that disturbed me. Rick called this "flooding." I've been told that flooding is a widely used clinical term; I had just not heard it before. Rick notes:

> This term 'flooding' is elegantly described by physician Claudia Osborn in *Over My Head*, her account of recovery from TBI after being hit by a car while riding her bicycle. Dr. Osborn gave many examples of flooding, often having to do with being so overloaded with stimuli and decisions to make that she just shut down and was unable to act. She describes the problem of trying to process too much information too quickly with the resulting failure at the task, and then the secondary emotional response of anger or tears.

He said that when a town floods, traffic can't get through the intersections. Our minds are like that. Between the excruciating challenge of wracking our brains trying to think of words, and observing ourselves on the verge of defeat, while our emotions are on the brink of falling apart, no wonder we flood.

Speech-language therapy is not like psychotherapy where it's a good thing to touch on emotion because you're unearthing something critical. When I flooded with Rick, he made clear that I needed to manage the flooding so I could function and perform the job at hand. So even today when I'm trying something hard, I take a deep breath and say to myself, "I have work to do. I can't flood." This means that I have to be alert to the dangers of pressing on. I have to be able to identify when my brain needs rest so I don't flood.

Speaking of water, one time he told me to use my cognitive energy like water in a dam, and channel it.

Cognitive strain or "burn"

Rick explained that the brain is different from muscles that develop after being torn down through exercise. The TBI survivor must avoid over-exercising her brain. We know when we have pushed our other muscles to the limit because we feel the "burn." It's similar with a brain injury. The awful cognitive "burn" (or "cognitive fatigue" or "cognitive strain") that we feel at, say, a noisy family celebration of a holiday, is a signal that we need to stop and rest. If you keep going, thinking you're being strong and persistent and brave, you can hinder the healing process. You can actually set back your recovery. Rick's practical advice like that has been invaluable.

Professionals and TBI survivors use the term "cognitive fatigue" a lot, but the word "fatigue" is too limited because it connotes simple tiredness. Normal people can be pretty unforgiving or completely clueless about the unique nature of brain fatigue. If a soldier in boot camp complains to his drill sergeant of fatigue, he'll be ridiculed and worse. I use the word only to compare it to the way a paperclip gets fatigued when you bend it back and forth. Eventually it snaps. Similarly, an injured brain "snaps" or "shuts down" when it's overloaded.

Other metaphors

My antennae are always up for new ways of describing various aspects of this injury.

Writing about Venice in his book *Watermark*, Joseph Brodsky says the fog can be so thick that if you go out on an errand you can find your way back "via the tunnel your body has burrowed in the fog; the tunnel is likely to stay open for half an hour." Memory is like that fog. You feel rushed to remember something because the fog is closing around the word or thought you're trying to see and express.

Because the injury is invisible and I "look great," I explain that even though I look the same, it's like my brain is in traction. I mentioned earlier that Rick Sanders' notes quoted me as saying that my brain feels as though it is sunburned and that everyday life is like the sun bearing down on it. This helps explains survivors' anti-social tendencies: if you're badly sunburned, you'll stay away from heat lamps and tanning booths. Similarly, we avoid noisy restaurants or overstaying dinner parties, even intimate ones.

As I've said, simple "fatigue" is inadequate to describe the cognitive fatigue or strain we feel. When friends ask me what that's like, I liken it to running the microwave and toaster at the same time, at least in our house – I blow out all the circuits and shut down. Sometimes I tell them it feels like a hangover, only it's a "cognitive hangover."

When I told Rick my term "cognitive hangover," he wrote:

I like that term. People can probably relate a bit to that. Also, it seems to me that there is some overlap with the kind of migraine where you need to lie down in a quiet room with the shades drawn. Maybe people could relate to that, too.

SLP testing

Our testing and cognitive work has been both fascinating and frustrating. "Speech-Language Pathologist" tells only a small part of what Rick does. He works with me on all things cognitive, all those things that I struggle with, like problem-solving, deductive reasoning, and pacing myself, as well as actual speech, sustaining a narrative, which falters when the topic is complicated or conceptual or mathematical or emotional or . . . well, lots of things.

We found that I struggle the most cognitively and in my speech when it's a "perfect storm" of something complex and emotionally charged, like "how have you been?", politics, the Middle East, the relative merits of Democrats and Republicans, or some of the more sophisticated interactions with people I love. And worst of all is when there's a time limit.

Earlier, I mentioned scoring high on one of Rick's tests. I knew what neuropsychologists call my "speed of processing" was slow, but the results didn't reflect that. When I got home I felt very blue and I had to go for a long walk. I wanted to take some tests that pinpointed my deficiencies; I wanted somehow to quantify my injury. Those came shortly thereafter. That was the day I remembered the verse, "and the Lord turned Job's captivity when he prayed for his friends." And so I walked in big circles in conservation land and prayed for my family and friends and colleagues, and I began to feel better.

I coined the term "residual intelligence." I didn't copyright it or publish it in a medical journal or anything; I just said it to Rick as something I have because I can still score high on some of the tests, like reading comprehension or guessing what shape comes next. Using the familiar metaphor, it was like my brain was in traction but I could still curl 40 pounds. Again, my problem with the results of those tests is that a high score says nothing about the cognitive strain and fatigue you have to fight through while you're taking them, not to mention the harsh fall you take afterwards.

Cognitive activities

Just as an MRI takes pictures of the brain from different angles, a wide variety of cognitive activities requires effort from different parts of the brain. They are both _diagnostic_ to help pinpoint specific limitations, and serve to _strengthen_ those areas when possible. Memory "muscles," for example, can be re-trained and strengthened. (Note: The muscle metaphor works in this instance, but as mentioned earlier, not if it's used to push a brain-injured patient to press on through discomfort, thinking the brain is like a "no pain, no gain" muscle.)

My favorite activity required both creativity and pure logic, and demonstrated for Rick the limitations of my cognitive clipboard. I had to use strategies to get through it, such as writing little clues to myself along the way.

In Speech-Language Pathology sessions we try and link cognitive activities to life in the real world; for example, "write down things you are likely to forget." But it's important to note this distinction: with this activity you can relax in knowing that the activity designer gives you all the information you need to solve the problem.

In the workplace, however, you are not at all guaranteed that people are giving you the right information. As a professional, you need to determine what information is missing and seek it out. In my brain-injured state, this would be embarrassing and humbling because of my new limitations. Realizing this made me aware of the sheer devastation of this injury.

Another activity featured Rick reading aloud a paragraph containing a specific number of "fact points." I would then try to recall as many of these as I could. The paragraph went something like this:

> As a woman went to the grocery store, her wallet fell out of her coat without her noticing. She did her shopping, and at the cashier noticed her wallet was missing. She put all of the groceries back and drove home. As she opened the front door, the phone rang and when she answered it a little girl said she had found the woman's wallet. The woman was relieved!

These are the kinds of things Rick and I worked on together:

- He taped me talking, and we listened to it together, noting when I began to stutter or blank out.

- He taped me reading a passage of text for two minutes and noted I did not have nearly the fluency problems as in a conversation.

- He presented me with a map of Washington D.C. and listed some of the attractions there. My task was to create a reasonable itinerary involving time and place for one eight-hour day.

- On the computer, I took 15 minutes and read ten pages about Mark Twain. (Topics of other reading comprehension activities included dental technological advances, hurricanes, Jules Verne and Apollo 11.) I then answered eight multiple-choice questions. We then repeated the activity six months later to see what, if anything, had changed.

This is the kind of homework Rick would give me:

- Think about what you can do under optimal conditions. What is the best environment for you? What is the worst?

- What support do you need from family and friends? What does "support" mean for you?*

- Tape a two-minute conversation with someone and bring it in; for example, read an article and summarize it, or tell someone about an important event in your life.

- It's important that people who are significant to you know how difficult this injury is. Consider how you might do that.**

- How many words can you think of to complete "head______"? (e.g., "headcount") How many words can you think of to complete "black______". (e.g., blackboard)

- Let's choose an article in a magazine. I want you to read it and then write a one-page summary of it.

- Prepare answers to this question: "What can I help you do, both now and over the next few weeks?"

- Imagine what you consider to be a good quality of life. That will help us figure out what we're aiming for. Describe a meaningful and satisfying life, and then we will discuss what is reasonable and possible.

- *(After 1 year of sessions)* At this point, what do you hope to accomplish next in our sessions?

- *(After two years of sessions)* List the things that rejuvenate you, and the things that drain you.

- Take 15 minutes to write, "What I will work on through December 31." *(this was mid-October of that year)*

* I said I had all the support I needed from my family, but I was stumped on what support I needed from friends. What does it mean to say, "I need my

friends to be there for me"? I said I enjoyed live music, playing music, going to a movie, sharing a glass of wine and one-on-one conversation. That was before I realized that going to a movie was excessive stimulation, and that I wasn't allowed to have any alcohol.

** I struggled with that because I didn't want their pity, and I didn't want to be seen as a complainer.

Strategies from Rick

- Rather than repeat a word, leave silence as you formulate your next thought verbally. Silence is less distracting to the listener than stuttering.

- Check out the Brain Injury Association of America for information and support at www.biausa.org.

- Make a draining activity like bill-paying or filing **time-based**, not based on whether you've completed it. In other words, think time-based, not task-based.

- It's not so much the number of activities you're doing; it's the nature of those activities.

- Avoid isolation! Go ahead and orchestrate time with a friend yourself if you have to.

- Prepare a script of a sentence or two to answer the inevitable question, "How are you?" Good examples include, "I'm making progress but I hear I have a long road ahead of me," and "Better thanks, but not 100 percent. How are things with you?"

- Also prepare a script for situations in which you need to defer a difficult conversation; for example, "Let me think about that and let's talk about it soon," and "That's a tough one to talk about right now. Do you have any time tomorrow?"

- In social settings, agree with your spouse on signals ahead of time; for example, "If I ask you if you're ready to go, that means I'm struggling." Think about how to expend your cognitive gas tank.

- One way to respond when someone asks about your work situation is to say, "It's upsetting to talk about it. I never expected to be out of work."

- Tell me about your dinner out with Lynne. Try not to stammer. Speak deliberately. (Note: I spoke carefully, pausing to consider my word choices instead of stammering, and I did pretty well.)

- Your strongest link is old information. Your weakest link is new information.

- You need to recalibrate your expectations. If you had not done so much on Wednesday night, you might not have needed so much down time on Thursday and Friday.

- Try to plan your rest times in advance. Schedule them the way you would any other important event.

- When preparing to read nonfiction, consider **S**, **Q** and **3R**: S for **Survey** (consider the length and complexity of the reading); Q for **Questions** (write down your questions on the reading as you go); and 3R for **Read, Recite** (say your answers out loud, or write them down next to your questions) and **Review** (look back on what you read)

- When undertaking a reading comprehension activity, summarize each page as you complete it. This technique is like rock climbing and setting a stake before going higher.

- Build in necessary time-outs. When you are working on something, set your alarm for 30 minutes, or 45 minutes, or an hour so that you do not lose track of time and overdo it.

- Your cognitive energy is like gas in the car. Keep your eye on the gas gauge. Periodically take ten-minute breaks. Get away from the task. Maybe take a walk outside.

- You need to take the load off of your working memory. You do this by verbalizing the problem you are struggling to solve in your head, and then writing it down.

- Prioritize the things you want to get done that are important to you, and look for ways of succeeding. Be sure to schedule them. Avoid the drain of perceived failure.

- One way to minimize what you put on your mental clipboard is to express the thing in words out loud. We call that "verbal mediation."

Miscellaneous interactions

- I told him I had a really hard time at the grocery store. He said that this didn't surprise him because they involve a lot of noise and decision-making, and are visually over-stimulating, what with scanning products and reading labels.

- I told him I sat on a plane before takeoff and found myself growing increasingly anxious and claustrophobic, which I had never felt on a plane before. He said that survivors can have increased anxiety because of first-hand experience that the world is not in our immediate control. This can cause some people to avoid going out in crowds or to just feel more at ease and safe staying at home.

- I told him some friends had said how great I was doing, and that I felt skeptical of their observations of progress because I'm experiencing my so-called recovery from the inside. He said their comments were valid and truthful. He also said that people want me to be better so that their world can be restored.

- I told him that I had to speak angrily to someone because this person had been drinking heavily and physically threatened one of my children. What surprised me was that I was crystal clear in my outburst, and Rick explained that emotionally charged situations can result in a survivor with speech problems speaking more fluently.

- It disturbed Rick that I would tell him I always felt like I was recovering from extreme cognitive exertion. That focused our attention on pacing and ways to relieve memory pressure on my mental clipboard.

- Two years into the injury, I was still expressing surprise about my harsh crash and recover cycles. Rick told me not to be surprised when I crash, and that I just had to realize I'm going to pay for my cognitive exertions. That's why I have to choose them wisely.

- He stated the simplest, most concise explanation for my new life: "You've had changes in how your brain processes information."

Throwing me a lifeline

A year and a half into the injury, when my hopes for recovery really started to flag, Rick told me he thought that I would continue to recover. I said something skeptical, and he said that he didn't think he could do what he does if he believed that his patients would not recover. Rick told me that in his practice he has followed many of his former patients and has seen them continue to progress over their lifetimes, including returning to competitive employment several years after the date of injury. In his calm and protective way, he threw me a lifeline.

Two years into the injury, he said, "The window is still open for you. You are still recovering."

SESSIONS WITH MY SOCIAL WORKER

"People that matter to you need to know how your life has been affected, and they learn that from you."

How Sally Johnson (MSW, LICSW) helped me

Seeing a social worker was one of the last things I ever thought I would need to do. I have always had a wonderful family, a strong marriage, great friends and a very good job. But a brain injury threatens all of that, and less than a year into my recovery, it became clear that I would benefit from seeing a social worker. Sally Johnson became an indispensible member of my recovery team.

What does "support" mean

Survivors often hear that support from family is critical in the recovery process. But the word "support" is vague, and the nature and extent of it varies from person to person. Sally was very good about helping me be clear about the specific support I need from my family. For example, I learned that I could tell them:

- "Rescue me when I am conversationally cornered at a social event."

- "When you see a taxing person pull into the driveway, tell me so I can retreat."

- "Be my forward scout and identify a restaurant that's quiet. This relieves me of being the bad guy in a noisy restaurant because I won't have to say I can't eat there and spoil the evening."

Making sure spouse's needs are being met

Just after Lynne's parents died within seven weeks of each other, Sally asked me what kind of support Lynne was getting. I realized that she was getting no professional support. She has me, of course, and her sister, and a few close friends, but even among us Lynne is a private person and keeps a lot inside. Sally asked how Lynne relieves stress, and I said I thought by reading and going to the gym. I added that she fights pervasive winter blues by knitting. She replied that these might be good outlets for her stress, but still I wondered whether she needed something more formal.

I encouraged Lynne to go with me the next time I met with Sally. Sally reminded us that TBI survivors can become self-absorbed, and not as focused as they should on the challenges of their spouse. She also reinforced the need for both of us to communicate clearly with each other, which would help clear up misunderstandings and misperceptions.

Asking great questions

Sally asked me one of the all-time great questions during this recovery process. I'd told her that I had written and delivered the eulogies on behalf of both of Lynne's parents, and she asked, "Were they the same eulogies you would have written before your injury?"

I laughed at the perfection of that question, and then I thought hard about it. I e-mailed her that the eulogies probably were the same eulogies as I would have written before the injury but that, 1) they carried with them the terrible cycle of crashing and recovering during the writing, 2) had taken me ten times longer to write, and 3) were ten times harder to write.

It struck me that in asking that question, Sally helped me learn something significant about my injury and the "me" wrapped up inside of it. I had not lost much of my insight or my feelings for those I loved, but communicating all of that had become a major struggle.

Sally asked another extremely probing question. Two years into the injury I got it into my head that I wanted to complete a particular project by mid-August. As much as I was able, I worked to complete it and drove myself into the ground. I more or less achieved my goal but I paid a huge price in the now familiar crash and recover cycle. When I recounted this to her, Sally asked point blank: "Why do you think you set mid-August as your deadline, knowing that would be a busy time with Chris and Andrew getting ready for college?" Her acute perception made me think about my relationship with my family and my work in fresh ways.

Providing invaluable perspective on recovery based on her vast experience

I told Sally about an unpleasant interaction I'd had with a doctor who I believed had misdiagnosed me, and she asked, "What are you looking for at this point in your recovery?" I said I wanted two things: 1) a straightforward, unambiguous acknowledgement that what happened to me the night of September 21, 2005, led to the classic sequelae of a brain injury; and 2) I wanted him to draw on his expertise working with other mild TBI survivors, the implication being he had no other patients like me.

Both of these were sticking points, points that stuck in my throat. As we continued talking, I told Sally, "as far as seeing a doctor who will somehow treat me and cure me, maybe I should instead focus on what I already know helps and hinders and try to improve the quality of my life." Her face sort of lit up in confirmation, and we talked further about having realistic expectations of what a doctor can do for someone with a mild TBI.

After our meeting, I decided to see a new doctor, and he did acknowledge my brain injury for what it was, and is. This conversation with Sally also led me to seek out additional help with coping strategies. After some research, I contacted Wayne A. Gordon at Mount Sinai Medical Center[33] and he told me about a three-month program that might be useful for me. I enrolled, and found that experience a critical part of the recovery and rehabilitation process, which will be the subject of another book.

Homework

This is the kind of homework Sally would give me:

- Give some serious thought to the psychological and emotional part of coping with family challenges, how you carve out time for yourself, and how you manage stress.

- List all of the things that have gotten better in the past three months.

Strategies

- People that matter to you need to know how your life has been affected, and they learn that from you.

- Your recovery from a brain injury is not a matter of your will to recover. You will get fatigued – although the word "fatigue" is an understatement – so you need to find ways to reduce the severity of your fatigue. For example, plan for down time, whether it is a nap or simply a break.

- It's important that you make choices in your daily activities. Try to learn to "put the ball down" rather than "drop the ball."

- Regarding how badly you feel so much of the time, don't think in terms of having a "bad day" and a "good day." Think of it as having a "better" or "worse" day. Start an "accomplishment" list, which will help you develop perspective on your progress.

- Consider all the factors that might go into having a better or worse day; for example, the weather, your physical surroundings, the amount of noise and visual stimulation, how much and intensely you interact with people.

- Have your spouse and others *help you* prevent bad crashes, but realize it is up to you to prevent them. Have them help you be moderate in your daily activities.

- Catch "terrible" before it happens. Pacing yourself throughout the day is critical. You can feel like you turn a corner in your recovery and then overdo it and regress. Calculate whether what you plan to do will be worth the inevitable crash.

- With a brain injury you can't always cite cause and effect for mid-day crashes. Some crashes are unpredictable. They can be for a variety of reasons, or for no reason. Often, nothing precipitates a crash, so be easy on yourself if you don't see a connection or pattern. If you do, try to plan differently next time; for example, plan fewer tasks or activities in a day. Pace yourself better.

- If necessary, just say, "I can't do this!" You can't be any clearer than that.

MOVING ON FROM APPOINTMENTS TO DAY-TO-DAY LIVING

It's time now to move from seeing professionals to doing what you do the most of: living your new life day-to-day. The next chapter takes a hard look at some of the social challenges someone with a brain injury faces, even when surrounded by loved ones.

18 – The Challenges of Social Interaction, and Crushing Loneliness

AVOIDING THE NEW NEIGHBOR

A big snow had fallen where I live in rural Massachusetts, and I headed for the quiet of nearby conservation land in the 11 degree cold. I walked to the end of our road and tramped across a field into a meadow, and from there to a little bridge across a frozen stream. I stood on the bridge, aware that this was the first winter in many years that I had taken the time to appreciate the way the snow draped the branches and caught the bright December light. The quiet sharpened the new ringing in my ears but I felt at peace. When I headed home through the drifted snow I still felt at peace.

Then I turned the bend on our road and spotted our new neighbor shoveling snow in his driveway. For four months I'd been meaning to stop by to introduce myself and welcome him to the neighborhood, but I hadn't had a day when my brain felt good enough to do it. I obviously couldn't walk by him now without saying anything, so this simple thing had become complicated.

He didn't see me, so I quickly walked back around the bend to the corner where I stood in the cold and brooded, weighing my options. Decision-making with a brain injury is no longer an automatic process. If I pressed on, I'd have to introduce myself and apologize for my failure to welcome him. I'd have to talk.

I didn't want to talk. I never *want* to talk. I wasn't feeling especially friendly or, God knows, articulate. No, meeting him now would be way too complicated and fraught with embarrassment. When I stammered I'd feel compelled to say, "Oh, that. I have a brain injury." I've found myself in too many conversational corners where I have felt compelled to explain my brain injury and have seen the uncertain look on people's faces. I see in their eyes or hear in their voices that they are trying to decide if I am mentally handicapped or even insane. Many times when the fact of my brain injury comes up, they start talking slower and simpler, as though to a child.

I didn't want to walk around the block and approach my house from the other direction because it would require a two-mile hike through heavy snow. That wasn't what I'd signed up for when I went out for a stroll. Plus, I didn't have my cell phone to call Lynne to explain why it was taking so long to get back.

I decided to wait him out. And so there I stood.

More time passed. I put too much thought into how I should act when a car drove past. Standing around by the side of the road doing nothing in the intense cold looked weird.

Thinking that it might be safe to approach the bend to listen for sounds of shoveling, I got closer and then closer, still out of my new neighbor's sight. I considered the possibility that he might simply be resting from shoveling, so I listened for other sounds of his presence.

Hearing nothing, I did something brave. I rounded the bend completely and walked past the foot of his driveway in full view. It was completely, blessedly shoveled from the road to his garage. I stood appreciating his work ethic, but mostly I appreciated his absence. I was emancipated! The knot in my stomach loosened, and I was free to walk the rest of the way home without having to interact with anybody!

I checked my watch. My indecision and my dread of social interaction were so overpowering that I had stood in the cold for an hour and a half. Yet most of the time, like the other TBI survivors you'll meet in this chapter, I am lonely.

THE CHALLENGES OF ONE-ON-ONE CONVERSATION

"Can't count the number of friends I've lost, can't count the number of days I've lost to exhaustion, can't count the number of events I missed or had to leave early, can't count the number of times I have had to put my ear plugs in, can't count the number of conversations I've avoided, can't count the number of times I've inadvertently offended friends, family, my wife. How can anyone put into words the social devastation and loneliness we've experienced?" Mike

One-on-one conversation can be almost as difficult as navigating a party. I hadn't seen my sister in a year or so, and she started telling me about some work-related problem. I wasn't tracking at all. I kept thinking, "Is she almost done?" I would nod and say "uh-huh" at all the parts requiring affirmation that I understood what she was talking about, but afterwards, I had absolutely no memory of a single thing she'd said. It was as if the part of my brain that used to let me fully engage with people had turned into a black hole that sucked in thought and trapped it.

Baseball season is a gift for me because it's a chance to avoid talking, especially when I need to recover from a social interaction. Four years into the injury, I was watching baseball at a friend's house. During a commercial, he started talking. In a mild panic I tried to find the mute button on his remote, but couldn't. He continued talking, and once again everything he said was sucked into my cranial black hole. I finally had to say, "I want to listen to you, but I can't listen to the TV and you at the same time. Sorry!"

The game was still on when my youngest son, who was working on his homework, asked us to define a few words. I knew them all, but that gravitational force was sucking energy from my brain because of the game on the TV, and because my fatherly pride made me want to respond to my son before my friend did. The time pressure made it impossible for me to formulate any response at all. I think most parents want to look good in front of their children – we want them to be as proud of us as we are of them – and it grieved me to falter in front of my son.

In an interview, Eric Clapton said he had decided to get sober after his son was born because he didn't want Conor to see him drunk. I thought hard about that decision after this and other seemingly trivial incidents with each of my sons. People with TBI hate it that their spouses and children see them brain injured, but we really don't have a choice. Survivors are living in and with a new reality. Lynne said I can count on our sons' basic goodness and compassion and love, and of course she's right about that. Still, people with TBI get tired of feeling like village idiots.

A man out standing in his field

Here is an analogy that has helped me think about and explain to others why TBI survivors find it easier to be alone. Even though we realize that this can lead to alienation, loneliness, and sometimes even depression, we believe it is preferable to what I call "the eternal tension of the shortstop."

Pretend you are watching a movie of a man standing in some grass. He's just standing there. The camera slowly backs up – or "pans out," if you want to get technical – and now you see the larger context; he is standing in a big field all alone. It is a very peaceful scene. A rabbit hops by.

The scene cuts and then opens onto the same man standing in the same grass. This time, as the camera backs up you see that he is playing shortstop in a baseball game, and the pitcher is going into his windup. The shortstop tenses up, crouches down, and starts hitting his glove with his fist, waiting for the batter to hit the ball. The batter might swing and miss, he might hit the ball in his direction, or might not even swing at all. But the shortstop has to be ready. The stakes are huge. You hear a crack of the bat, and the shortstop suddenly lunges toward the ball, catches it, and throws the batter out at first base. He has succeeded this time, but the episode has taken its toll.

When a survivor is alone, he is the man in the first field. Nobody expects anything from him, there is nothing for him to respond to, and he is not at all tense. If he is not quite at peace, he is at least focused on what his injury is demanding of him or denying him. When a survivor is with other people, however, even with one other person, he can feel a lot like a shortstop, waiting for a conversational ball to head in his direction. Maybe it will be a line drive, or just a lazy few hops, or a bunt to run in for. Regardless of whether the batter even hits the ball, the shortstop is in a perpetual state of tension, waiting to react to a possible hit.

All this is to say that being with another person, with the possible exception of another survivor – with whom occasional confusion and silence is expected – can be quite draining. Survivors have a hard time weighing things like facial expressions, a speaker's intention or tone of voice, and whether we've said too much or too little. Stress and anxiety increase, of course, with the passage of time because we overload with information quickly, and many times we're thinking – or praying – "How do I extract myself from this situation?"

The shortstop is looking over at the dugout, trying to signal to the manager to take him out of the game. Unable to catch the manager's attention, he lies down between second and third base and closes his eyes. The shortstop – and this metaphor – grew tired. Spectators head for the exits, and you, the reader, turn the page.

THE SOCIAL-LIFE VANISHING ACT

Tom and Arthur

Before the accident Tom and Arthur (Chapter 2) were "very social." They had a lot of friends, enjoyed parties and dinner engagements, and "loved to be with people." After the accident "people who we thought were our friends, they said, call us when it's over with. We can't handle this."

Tom's sudden and unpredictable panic attacks created almost insurmountable obstacles to a social life:

> Arthur and I were having a great time at the beach in Maine. We used to go on vacation in Maine all the time when I was a kid, so I loved it. We settled in to a great hotel and when one of our girlfriends showed up the three of us walked to a restaurant for lunch. I began to feel closed in inside the restaurant. Our meals arrived, I took one bite, and I got so anxious I had to excuse myself. I went to the men's room and saw in the mirror I was white as a ghost. I felt nauseous and went outside.

> That was it. For the rest of our vacation I was completely out of commission with vomiting, night sweats, and cold sweats during the day. My anxiety is totally unpredictable; it can soar in a second. Even when I'm in a happy mood it can kick in and take over my whole body and soul. You don't have to be in a bad mood or have something go wrong. I could go for a walk and feel good and then just flip for no reason. You can't imagine how hard it is to be around people when anxiety so intense can all of a sudden just jump you.

Saying goodbye to who we were

My friend Elizabeth puts it this way:

> This is not a life-changing event . . . This is a whole new life. Just as
> an infant is fragile, naked and unsure of its new environment, so am I.
> The hardest part is saying goodbye to who I was . . . and those who
> knew her.
>
> How do you explain to friends and loved ones that you're not who
> they've known for 32 years . . . even though you look the same –
> strong and healthy? If you choose not to explain it, even to colleagues,
> what do you say when your behavior is suddenly different? Or if they
> catch errors of cognitive deficit? What if you can't deal with their
> frustration because you are suddenly millions of miles away, lost in the
> question of "What's happening to me?"

Gregg and Diana's (Chapter 2) relationships with friends have changed as well.
They discovered that they can keep the friends who understand Gregg's injury,
but have lost some friends "who just don't understand it":

> We have a close friend and as much as we like him, we can't have
> much to do with him anymore only because he's such a talker. He's
> very vivid and can see when Gregg's overwhelmed and he lowers his
> voice, but keeps talking. Other people who don't get the injury avoid
> Gregg. I'd say the friends we have now are the people who really
> understand the injury and can read Gregg pretty well. We've made a
> lot of new friends through brain injury groups and they are supportive.
> I also get a lot of personal support from my co-workers.

Reflecting this theme of social avoidance simply because it's easier, one low
day I wrote in my journal:

> After my family there's a sharp drop-off in cognitive investment. My
> social needs have been co-opted by the devastation I experience after
> spending time with friends. While I need even my closest friends in

varying degrees, I guess I'd prefer them to remember me the way I was, rather than the sliver I let them see, and not burden them OR ME with the aftermath.

I'm not sure if I was fooling myself because how long or how well could we live without close friends? Many times Lynne and I will be getting ready to go out for the evening with friends and I just don't feel up to it. I will be tugging on my socks thinking, "Everyone will have a lot more fun without me there." Usually she talks me down from the ledge, we see our friends, and I'm always reminded how sweet, generous and fun they all are.

One evening we were expecting four friends over for dinner and, knowing I was having a rough day, Chris asked me, "Are you looking forward to tonight?" Without thinking how it would sound, I said, "No. I have no social needs. In fact, I have anti-social needs." As it turned out, once they arrived we shared a lot of laughs that evening.

Clearly, who we were doesn't exist anymore, only who we are. And who we are now is not who we ever expected or wanted to be. But we must remember that our friends and our family love us, and no less an authority than the Bible tells us to "love your neighbor as yourself." This is not a life-affirming injury so we must keep always before us reasons to affirm life. More on that in the final chapter.

People might find it easier to avoid us

"Expect to be surprised by who you hear from and who you don't hear from, or by who fails to greet you on the street or in a store." Gregg

". . . my neighbors find me burdensome, my friends shudder at me; when they see me on the street they turn away quickly. Like the dead I have passed out of mind; I have become like some article thrown away." Psalm 31:11-12

TBI survivors aren't the only ones who go out of our way to avoid people. We learn quickly that some people find it easier to avoid us, too. As hurtful as it is to see happen, Gregg observed, "It's the same if you have cancer. It's not that people are being mean-spirited. It's that people don't know what to say and they are nervous. It's easier to avoid the situation." Gregg continued:

> I was always the type to call people up when they had a tragedy although my parents would say, don't disturb them. But even if somebody has died, you're not bothering them. They want to talk and they'll let you know if they don't want to talk. I think you can expect that a certain number of people will totally try to avoid you when you have a traumatic brain injury.
>
> I noticed [a relative] slip into the other room without addressing me…I was in the kitchen and he slipped past me as fast as he could…In the grocery store you can tell people are trying to avoid seeing you. You know they've seen you, but they slip into another aisle. A friend, a motorcycle cop, he used to stop over right after my injury, but ever since then he drives down my street and sees me in the driveway and just keeps driving. So he's totally avoiding me now.

As part of a panel discussion at Boston University with a few other survivors, we talked about the waxing and waning of friendships post-injury. A few of us shared stories of how hard it is to sustain friendships with certain people – maybe they are too loud, too self-absorbed, too draining – and I spontaneously waved my hand toward the panel whom I had just met an hour before and I said, "These are my friends." Such is the bond we share in the injury.

You might find the need to cultivate new friends who understand the effects of the injury. Tom's partner Arthur wrote to me:

> Some friends told us we were "too high maintenance" as a result of Tom's injury and asked us to "get in touch when Tom was better." (Needless to say, we decided that they weren't true friends.) We were saddened by the intolerance of people we thought were our friends, but we learned to move on. If you can find other people who have been through similar trauma, they can be a great resource and be more understanding.

Friendship, or mere compatibility?

I had a very close friend, closer to me even than my brother. Two full years after the accident it occurred to me that he had never called or visited me, even though he lives nearby. Thinking it was self-centered of me even to wonder, I asked Lynne if she could think of anything he had done for me since the accident, and neither of us could think of a thing.

I had to ask myself a hard question: Are we friends? Have we ever been friends? I'd always assumed we were exceptionally close because we shared so many interests and frames of reference and had a lot of laughs and many deep, late-night conversations. But my jaw-dropping realization was that this was mere compatibility. It was not true friendship.

I took comfort from the Psalms. My friend had failed to reach out to me, but Psalm 27: 5-8 offered assurances that God's hand is on me. I could find rest in God's love:

> For in the time of trouble He shall hide me in His pavilion; in the secret of His tabernacle shall He hide me; He shall set me up upon a rock. I had fainted: unless I had believed to see the goodness of the Lord in the land of the living. Wait on the Lord; be of good courage, and He shall strengthen thine heart: wait, I say, on the Lord.

"Surviving the holidays"

"The loneliest I feel is in a roomful of normal people." Brain injury support-group member

I received an invitation to a brain injury support meeting weeks before Thanksgiving. The topic was "Surviving the Holidays." Well, that's kind of negative, I thought. I soon found out why the meeting was focused that way, and why so many brain injury survivors find the holidays difficult.

Before my brain injury, I always looked forward to the big family gatherings around our Thanksgiving table. But four years into my injury, when we celebrated at the home of some of our closest friends, my feelings of isolation and aloneness intensified.

Our friends are aware of my limitations, but on this Thanksgiving I felt as though I had been thrust into a hostile environment. My family and close friends have figured out how to make social events as much a pleasure for me as it is for them by agreeing to stick to one conversation at a time. As Mike observed, trying to take in multiple conversations "is like somebody has an industrial fire hose and they're blasting you in the face."

Throughout the feast, four or five loud and simultaneous conversations forced me to keep getting up to leave the room. Of course, everybody was simply caught up in the moment, but besides the hostile-to-my-brain environment, I felt abandoned and unimportant. The many TBI survivors I have met report the same experiences.

On the day before Thanksgiving, Mike and I exchanged e-mails. We each expressed the hope that the day would turn out to be a good one for everybody. Yet it turned out that Mike was to have a Thanksgiving Day as unhappy as mine. We began texting from backrooms in the homes of our hosts:

> <u>Me</u>: Had injury 4 years so why is Thanksgiving so loud? You too?
>
> <u>Mike</u>: Hiding out right now. feel like a freak. guess we got to try and tuff it out. god knows we will pay tomorrow. good luck brother.
>
> <u>Me</u>: You too. In other room too. Whats kind of weird is nobody is saying "let's have one conversation bcz it's hard 4 John." Oh well, don't miss me too much guys!
>
> <u>Mike</u>: Yup I feel your pain. Gonna force myself to gym tomorrow. think it will help.
>
> <u>Me</u>: Hearing everyone laughing . . . makes u think "what can be so funny?"

Picture our situation. Here we are, two guys with TBI who are reluctant to leave our friends and families, but are so overwhelmed by multiple conversations and noise at our respective gatherings that we each retreat to rooms where we can text our grievances to each other, knowing we understand each other completely. And both Mike and I know the price we will pay tomorrow.

When I described this for Rick Sanders, he wrote:

> This is the sort of thing we address in our Family Strategies group, trying to educate spouse and relatives on how the TBI individual can still participate, perhaps by having one-on-one conversations out on the porch, and then returning briefly to the punch-bowl room to meet up with another conversational partner.
>
> When family is aware of this strategy it allows the survivor to participate. It alleviates loneliness to some degree for two reasons: directly because interaction is facilitated, and indirectly but, perhaps as important, the TBI person knows that others understand when they make the effort to change interactions in this way.
>
> These family gatherings are universal and these changes have a lasting healing effect. This is not to say all will be as before. That is often unrealistic. But it can be better, even good.

Stimulus overload

"Wanting to leave is essentially a coping mechanism. It's a survival strategy, not a behavioral problem." Barbara Webster

"It's the overstimulation, lights, and noise and conversation that are so hard," explains Gregg's wife, Diana. "It's amazing how fast Gregg can deteriorate in that kind of environment":

> Eating out in a restaurant can be pure torture for Gregg, especially if there are a lot of people in the room talking. On the few occasions when we want to eat out, we'll go very early, at 4 or 5 o'clock, and we call ahead of time to try to reserve a quiet corner. But forget it if the restaurant is echo-y and sound reverberates. It makes Gregg sick.

"Do I suffer consequences from social interaction?" Gregg asks the question rhetorically and answers it:

> 100 percent yes. What it feels like is hard to explain. My head feels horrible and headache-y and I want to lie down. Also I need total quiet in darkness. I feel sort of like I did when I first got the injury. The symptoms can last from an hour to an entire day. I can't do anything. It's like when you're so sick you just lie there and suffer. It's not like you're sleeping. You feel ill and you just want to lie there because you cannot do anything. It puts me in a catatonic state. I'm unable to answer questions or interact at all.

Not only is it hard to convey what our Thanksgiving Day or restaurant environments make us feel like, our normal appearance – no neck brace or body cast – does not exactly cry out for empathy. Barbara Webster (Chapter 10), a TBI survivor and support group leader, offers a valuable insight into the effects of such an environment on a survivor:

> A survivor may become difficult in a noisy, confusing social situation and the family and friends think he is being uncooperative, selfish, attention seeking or even exhibiting "behavioral problems." But the reality is that the environment is causing him to experience stimulus overload due to sensory hypersensitivities from his brain injury. Wanting to leave is essentially a coping mechanism. It's a survival strategy, not a behavioral problem.

Barbara's strategies

- **Listen:** I like to remember that everyone likes to be listened to and focus more on being a good listener.

- **Arrange a retreat place:** I always try to have a quiet place where I can take a break.

- **Plan ahead:** I don't plan to stay long when I know it may become overwhelming. I make sure I have easy days before and after big events.

- **Choose the margins:** Sometimes it helps to find a task to help with like serving or taking photos, to give you an excuse to stay on the outskirts.

THE COST OF SOCIAL AVOIDANCE: CRUSHING LONELINESS

"Nobody on the face of the earth, no doctor, therapist, or rehab person knows what it's like to be affected by TBI. They know only what their patients report and what their textbooks say. Loneliness? It's so lonely there should be another word for it." Mike

Mike confronts his new life: "You're in survival mode"

People with TBI feel powerful but contradictory impulses. We miss being with people, yet we dread it because we pay for even a simple evening in the home of friends. The cost is an array of brutal mental and physical miseries that I refer to collectively as "cognitive hangover."

Mike often hears from some of his friends, "I didn't invite you because you like to stay home." Sometimes when the phone rings and Mike's wife answers he hears her say, "Mike would never be able to do that. Don't bother asking him, he'll just get upset." The truth is that Mike would like very much to be able to do that, but usually it's just too hard. Sometimes it's impossible.

Getting ready to go out

Mike had been looking forward to an evening out with his best friends, but even before he headed out to meet them he was in, as he put it, "exhaustion mode," already feeling that terrible cognitive fatigue. He lay down for awhile, hoping some quiet would rejuvenate him, but he knew he couldn't manage the get-together. Mike told his wife he just couldn't go:

> She kept saying, "Why don't you let me drive you?" She was so persistent that I finally had to yell to make her understand. I know she wanted the best for me, but what happens is that people get it and yet they really don't get it. Her persistence suggested to me that it was a choice I was making, and it's not a choice. If choice was any part of it

I'd have spent the evening with my friends, but I was facing a physical barrier.

Before my injury I worked really long hours, I had circles of friends I kept in touch with regularly, and I was out every weekend. But that physical barrier is as if a person ran a marathon and took the SATs and three other exams all in the same day without any sleep and the next day your brain just doesn't work. You're in survival mode. Your brain just can't take in anything else.

Losing friends

Mike says that the only real friends he has now are the friends he has had since he was a kid. These are people who felt close enough to him that they were able to say after his accident, "Hey Mike, you know you're stuttering?"

After his TBI, Mike began to lose other friends. He attributes this to his expectation of recovering fully – "I was told I was gonna get better and most people do" – and so in the first year after the injury he "wasn't running around telling everybody that I have this injury because in my mind I'm convinced I'm gonna get better." In the second year it was the same thing. He didn't tell friends what was going on – "Why spread this miserable news?" – so over time he lost touch with more and more people.

Another reason Mike's friendships dried up was that they would e-mail him and leave voicemails, and he would just let the messages pile up. Mike had lost the ability to sort through the levels of urgency, so he would put off responding. Sometimes, he said, there might be 15 messages, and the sheer volume of messages so overwhelmed him that he would delete them all without reading or listening to them.

"What happens is all your friends, they are communicating, or they think they are communicating, but you can't communicate back." Mike's friends thought he didn't care enough to get back to them and Mike was so caught up in dealing with his injury that he didn't take the time to explain himself.

How do you prepare for loneliness?

Nobody in the medical community prepared Mike for the loneliness:

> Everyone I know with TBI is affected this way, so why doesn't anybody in the health care professions say that this happens to people? If you knew about this ahead of time, maybe you could deal with it better? Nobody tells you or warns you to help you watch out for it and deal with it. It's because nobody on the face of the earth, no doctor, therapist, or rehab person knows what it's like to be affected by TBI. They know only what their patients report and what their textbooks say.
>
> If you were blind, you'd be provided with a seeing-eye dog. TBI is an injury that causes social isolation and loneliness. Why is there no dog therapy for people with TBI? How can this be? If it wasn't for the soldiers coming back with this injury from Iraq and Afghanistan, nobody would talk about TBI at all. My God, what would happen if you got this injury thirty or forty years ago?

Men especially, I think, do not like to admit to loneliness. We like to think of ourselves as rocks, perhaps even as islands. But a brain injury strips all of that self-reliance away and bares our very human need for contact, and through contact, support.

Mike and I feel free to admit these intense feelings to each other. We can say to each other, "I know exactly how you feel." Nobody else can really say that to us, other than another survivor.

A harsh choice

Those of us living with TBI long for deep connections with other people, especially with our loved ones. But TBI punishes you with its low-level plateaus, demoralizing collapses and partial recoveries. If we choose to be with friends, we know that we will have to live for many hours and sometimes days with a cognitive hangover. If we choose to avoid people, we have to live with a loneliness that can be crushing. "Loneliness?" Mike said to me:

> It's so lonely there should be another word for it. I was thinking the other day that it's been almost two years since I have looked anyone in the eye. How lonely you feel without eye contact! I had no idea a person was able to feel this lonely.

My friend Elizabeth drew it this way:

Figure 8: Survivor Art

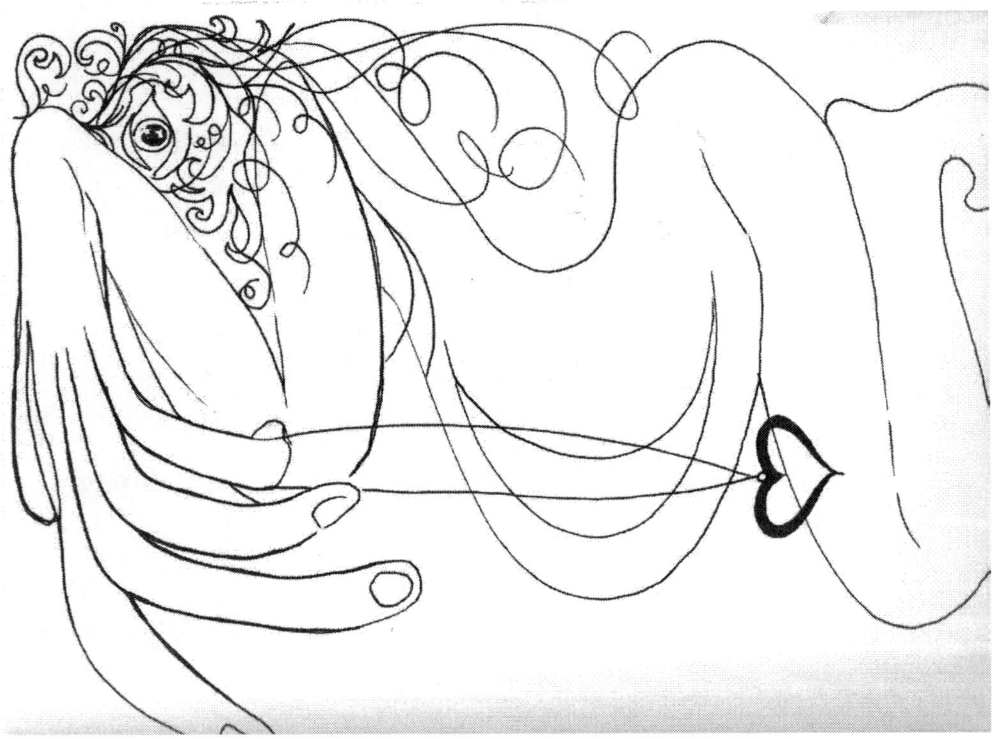

Artwork: Elizabeth Thyng Montanaro

Rick Sanders responds

After reading a draft of this chapter, Rick wrote:

> It is distressing to hear of Mike's experiences. Regarding loneliness, I
> have been showing my BU class on TBI a 1982 film entitled "Broken
> Rhymes," in which the UK researcher Neil Brooks says that the
> number one symptom that plagues survivors after other symptoms
> have been resolved is social isolation, loneliness. We try to prepare
> patients and families for this probability, mentioning support groups,
> making connections with other patients.

One of Mike's strategies

One of Mike's strategies is to let others know you're injured. He explains:

> When I was 100 percent certain that I would recover I tried to hide my
> injury from friends and that contributed to my loneliness. If I could
> live through that time again, I'd do it differently and ask for support.
>
> The only thing your social network knows is that you're not showing
> up or responding to e-mails and v-mails.
>
> Communicate to every important person in your life that you've got
> TBI, and ask someone you trust to provide the details to your network.
> If people in your network don't know what's happened to you, they
> can't support you.

Even though postcards from TBI Land are not the same as being there, trying
to explain what the injury is like is important. When it becomes too frustrating,
some survivors find it simpler to retreat. One friend observed that "most people
are ignorant about brain injury. When I stopped trying to explain it and
expecting them to understand I stopped being frustrated and disappointed that
they couldn't understand."

So some days you will try and explain and other days it will be too hard.

Suggestion: Ask friends questions

Having touched on this painful aspect of living with a TBI, one of the most important things I've learned is that the injury can be so consuming that survivors think of little else. Friends and loved ones of survivors are sure to notice this! After one survivor spent a full 15 minutes telling a graduate school class about nearly every aspect of his accident and his injury, he then said that none of his friends visited him anymore. Well, if this is all he talks about, of course people are going to start leaving him alone.

Time with friends should not turn into monologues. Remember what it takes to make a genuine connection with people. People don't want to be an audience. Survivors must remember to display normal codes of social niceties, and that includes asking questions. This also diverts draining attention away from trying to explain something that is extremely hard to explain and friends aren't likely to grasp anyway.

If you are with a friend, ask about work, family, other friends, hobbies, anything that the friend enjoys talking about. This sounds simple, but survivors should work hard at being at least pleasant and engaging to be with.

This is a good segue into strategies for surviving social minefields.

19 – Strategies for Surviving Social Minefields

I have been accumulating great strategies after working with my SLP Rick Sanders and Social Worker Sally Johnson. I share full credit with them. They each have about 25 years experience working with TBI survivors, and many a lot worse off than me. I have understood each tip they have given me, but I have also ignored or underestimated their importance.

Remembering to follow survival tips is probably the most important thing you can do to live better with even a mild brain injury. Many of them might not feel natural, so you have to consciously remember to put them into practice.

Strategy	Example
Agree on a coping signal with your spouse or partner	Use a word or phrase to signal a spouse or friend that you are finding it impossible to cope in a social situation. Whisper the signal and leave the room. He or she will provide you cover. My own signal is simple: I say to Lynne, *"I can't do this."*
Don't do the linger!	"I can't do the linger" sounds like a line from a Seinfeld script, but it's a tactic that works. After an event that requires your attendance, avoid the schmoozing that generally follows. Even before you begin to sag cognitively, flee.
Manage yourself at family and friend gatherings	It's usually easier to go into the kitchen before dessert and do all the pots and pans – with earplugs – than continue in conversation around the table. If someone comes out to help you, thank them and say that it's easier for you than talking. Your guest will probably understand.
Recognize what kind of day it is, and act accordingly	One day I wrote in my journal, "Told Lynne I felt handicapped today. Everything is hard." Both she and I knew I'd be keeping a very low profile all day.

Strategy	Example
Leave at the height of the party, when you're feeling good	Lynne and I went to a party with some close friends. Michael and Nancy Jane sang professionally early in their careers, and out came the show tunes on their grand piano. At one point, Michael and I launched into "My Funny Valentine," one part Sinatra (him) and one part Elvis Costello (me). When we nailed the ending we all laughed, Michael and I hugged, and I was happy. I immediately retreated upstairs and stretched out on a couch, not sleeping, just closing my eyes and enjoying the sounds of my dear friends laughing. I liked to think that they would be laughing harder had I been my old self, but that was okay. We'd had our moment. (Contrast this with my Thanksgiving experience, where I resented sitting in a back room. It marks the difference between "Adjustment" and "Acceptance.")
Say no to cruel traps!	Bumper stickers reduce complicated issues to a few words. Here in Massachusetts, one bumper sticker promoted a ban on certain animal traps and the catchy phrase turned out to be a valuable tool for me. If I'm confronted with the possibility of a cognitively draining experience I think, "Say no to cruel traps!" In a room where, say, multiple conversations are taking place, if somebody strikes up a conversation with you, *Say no to cruel traps* and excuse yourself.
Keep track of the time	Lynne asked if I wanted to go with her and Will someplace and I said sure. Then I counted how long it had been since I'd rested and it had been 5 ½ hours. I was due to crash and they went without me. I slept for two hours and was okay for the rest of the evening.
Have a friend keep an eye on the clock for you	Forty minutes into lunch with my friend Ted, I began slurring my words and it was getting harder for me to put my thoughts together. Like a good friend, Ted took the initiative and said we should probably wrap up. I saw that was a great strategy.34

Strategy	Example
Have somebody look out for you	Towards the end of a pretty busy day I thought I could do one more task, but Lynne looked out for me. I told her I would go to the grocery store, and she asked, "Are you sure you're up for that?" I thought about it and realized she was right. Another day I told her, "I feel okay today," and she urged caution and told me not to overdo it.
Keep track of your environment	One afternoon a friend of mine called and I picked up even though I knew it meant a conversation. As we got rolling – he's a good storyteller and we both laugh a lot – Will asked if he could plug his guitar in and play. I said sure. So I'm hearing about the time he learned to fly a helicopter, but I found really quickly that I was paying extra close attention because I was listening over Will's playing. As I paced the living room floor I could feel my cognitive battery wearing down. I got off the phone as soon as I could. I should have asked Will to wait until I got off the phone.
Be honest with your friends	Some people, even a lot of people, will not understand your injury. All the survivors in this book have friends who still "don't get it." I've learned that in the long run it pays to be honest and open with people, despite the short-term puzzlement on their faces or my own feelings of humiliation.

The lesson for the TBI survivor is to understand your injury. You will have to go through a lot of trial and error to find out your limits *and* your coping strategies.

20 – Support Groups and Volunteering: Yea or Nay?

SUPPORT GROUPS

They might become a crucial part of your recovery team

I gradually began to think of our local brain-injury support group as part of my recovery team, and participating in one, at some point, will likely benefit you. Some support groups include only survivors, some are limited to caregivers and friends of survivors, while others include both survivors and caregivers.

Potential benefits

The group I attend when I am able to get there is wonderfully supportive, and works the way a good support group should: offering each other advice and strategies that we've learned along the way. We can talk in a kind of shorthand to each other, the way combat veterans do, and in fact my friend Jim refers to people who do not have a brain injury as "civilians."

Another way of thinking of support groups is that we are prisoners tapping on the walls of our shared injury to each other, understanding and being understood. We do not try and hide our injury from each other the way we might with others, which sets the tone of honesty in our sessions. The kinds of strategies we share with each other range from preparing a shopping list for the grocery store to medical professionals we have benefited and learned the most from.

One support-group leader guide describes the essence of support groups as:

> . . . To help each other during extraordinary times within a nurturing environment. Personal expression and mutual support are the seeds of the group; increased coping skills and healing are the fruits.

Barbara Webster, long-time facilitator for the Framingham, MA support group in which I occasionally participate, finds that the two most important benefits for members continue to be:

- Connecting with others who really understand what you are going through, and

- Connecting with the right resources.

Despite great strides in recent years in research and in raising awareness, brain injury is a specialty in the healthcare field and finding the right specialists and resources can make all the difference. Barbara's right: a good support group will help survivors find access to these resources.

Barbara developed a support-group leader guide for the Brain Injury Association of Massachusetts for their support group leaders, adapting the national Brain Injury Association guide: *Helping Ourselves, A Guide for Brain Injury Support Groups*. The following pages contain an excerpt.

Benefits of Support Groups

Benefits	Why
Decreases feelings of isolation	Many survivors and family members often feel they have no one to turn to that understands how they feel or what they are going through, and a support group provides them with a place where they are not alone.
Encourages the sharing of similar experiences	This helps members feel less isolated and more empowered to deal with daily challenges.
Promotes emotional healing	Interpersonal contact is therapeutic.
Provides encouragement	Learning about the achievements of others who have overcome similar difficulties inspires the survivor to keep trying.
Creates environment that allows support group members to feel useful	They can use their knowledge and experience to benefit others, which is very satisfying.
Educates participants	The education is both formal and informal, from shared experiences to scheduled speakers providing members with specific information about various topics affecting their lives.
Provides a forum for the dissemination of information	Participants can learn about Brain Injury Association (BIA) activities throughout the state.
Enhances self-confidence and social skills.	Participants can develop and maintain important new connections.

Benefits of Support Groups, cont'd

Benefits	Why
Builds confidence	As members contribute to the group and work on problems they all have in common they grow more self-assured.
Provides a sense of safety	Support groups are confidential, supportive and non-judgmental so participants feel secure about expressing themselves.
Creates a sense of hope	As members discover they are not alone and realize that others in similar situations have healed and progressed over time, they are encouraged.
Generates growth	As long-term members see new participants and reminisce about where they began and how far they have come, they are encouraged and new participants are inspired.

Rick Sanders comments:

> These are great to show all that a good support group can do. Many people have a bias against groups with "support" in their names because they think it will just be a bunch of people whining about their problems. A good support group does listen to the everyday challenges members face, but will then be pro-active to help make it better. And there is solace, comfort, resolve and energy in knowing that someone has been through something similar and therefore really does understand you.

Warning . . .

However, think twice about attending a support group *early* in your recovery. Support groups should come with a warning, like on a pack of cigarettes. In the first year of my injury, I wasn't strong enough to hear these sad outcomes, not to mention saying anything at all constructive or useful, not while I felt so vulnerable and needy myself.

I needed nurturing and encouragement, but because everyone's injury was worse than mine, I felt I had to try to offer support. I was too vulnerable, frightened, and ignorant about mild TBI in general and my own mild TBI in particular to reach out to others. I left the group absolutely depleted, vowing never to go back.

Meeting long-time TBI survivors during your first year of recovery can be demoralizing because:

- Their personal stories might be a lot worse than your own and seriously depress you

- Their partners might be in the process of divorcing them and this might frighten you

- Their injuries might have occurred years ago and their failure to recover might scare you

Rick Sanders further observes:

> Some people do get a lot out of such groups midway or later in their first year. Excellent tips though, especially if the spouse or family member also comes. Sometimes they will have a broader perspective. The danger, or course, is that it can be disheartening to meet other families who are still dealing with a lot of disability years post onset.

At a minimum, create a two-person support group

One of the themes of this book is that, as a TBI survivor, you are not alone. Nobody likes to hear that somebody else is suffering, but most survivors do immediately feel a deep kinship when they hear other survivors' stories of life inside their injury.

The first time I met Mike (Chapter 2), we talked in the lobby at Spaulding Rehabilitation Hospital for about 40 minutes. Toward the end of that conversation, he told me that after living with the injury for over a year, I was the first person he had spoken to who also had a TBI. As we said goodbye until next time, we both felt a tight bond between us, as though we were combat veterans. From the time I first met him, I felt as though Mike needed me because I had been injured longer and my injuries not quite as severe. I felt I was and needed to be the strong one in our two-man support group.

We spoke, e-mailed and texted many times after that, and then for about two months he went silent. I didn't know that he was simply deleting all of his phone messages and all of his e-mail. As the time dragged on, I persisted in trying every way I knew how to get back in touch with him. I called his lawyer, wrote to his wife, and called his business partner. Nobody could or would tell me where Mike was. Obviously, I grew really worried about him. I kept thinking, "Don't leave us, Mike! Call me. You can tell me anything. I want to be here for you."

One day I was having an especially hard time and I felt more alone than ever. It suddenly hit me that Mike's absence was affecting me way more than I thought. I share certain sequelae with many of my survivor friends, but Mike and I shared the most. It was then that I realized that I needed Mike at least as much as he needed me. Only Mike understood how badly I felt every single day. And if he's drifted off into the ocean, where does that leave me?

It's great if we can be strong for someone else, but we need to realize, too, that we need to lean on another survivor from time to time. We need each other. After Mike returned to the land of the living and explained the situation (Chapter 18), we resumed our communications and friendship. Some months later I texted him about a bad day I was having because I knew he – of all people – would understand. He wrote back right away:

> Hang in there brother. I can't do this by myself, but no it's not going away. We have to stick together. Call me if you want to talk.

We did talk, and we continue to talk, and we continue to try and lighten the other's burden when we can. It is a deep friendship.

I went back when I was ready

A year or so later I went back to the group and was glad I did. I was starting to come to terms with the possible permanency of my injury, and I find the fraternity – and sorority – of other survivors to be of some comfort. I also felt I had something to contribute to this little community. I'd learned some valuable lessons that I was happy to share with them, and they with me. For example, one survivor compared the challenge of thinking and speaking, saying "It's like running on ice," and that image helped me.

Support groups aren't for everyone, but everyone needs support. If you already have a strong support system in place – family, friends, a community such as a church or temple – you might not benefit from a support group early on. However, if your recovery is slow, you will find that, in the words of the old spiritual, "nobody knows the trouble I've seen" . . . except a fellow TBI survivor.

Sometimes, support groups are most helpful if you were not diagnosed initially after an accident, or if lingering effects now interfere with your life and you are struggling to find help. Often they are most useful when formal rehabilitation is over but the lifelong rehabilitation process is not. They help fill the void.

"Silly hat day"

One support-group meeting I attended hosted a "silly hat day." I'd half remembered the event as I was leaving the house but I resisted the whole idea. The last thing I wanted to do was wear a silly hat. I'd seen Disney's Hunchback of Notre Dame and remembered that scene where they crown him the King of Fools. I already felt like the King of Fools and I didn't feel like wearing a silly hat to draw more attention to the fact.

Plus, it was "bring a funny story about your injury" day. I asked Lynne before I left the house, "Has anything funny happened because of the injury?" and she agreed that no, nothing funny had happened.

I didn't want to go empty-handed so I did bring a story to read – "Avoiding the New Neighbor" from Chapter 18 – and it went over pretty well. I learned that often the benefits of attending the group outweigh any awkwardness in playing along with things you might not be in the mood for.

Try different support groups

Barbara Webster says to try different support groups. The support group experience will vary depending on:

- The composition of the group at a given meeting;

- The timing in the rehabilitation process for the individual;

- The absence or presence of other supports in your life.

Sometimes one might strive to be seen as his/her "old helper self" and not receive the needed support. Sometimes there might be some denial and shock; for example, if you are the mildest of the mild TBI survivors present, you might think, "Is this really my new peer group?" A good facilitator will recognize all of this, and work at successfully incorporating new members in to the group.

Keep in mind that while support groups can be very therapeutic, they are not therapy groups. Many members will need to participate in therapy or counseling in addition to a support group.

Try different support groups if the first one doesn't feel right. Revisit the support group possibility if you find you didn't feel ready at your first attempt.

VOLUNTEERING

There are always going to be volunteer activities with which you can get involved. But they don't have to be done by you if they are now outside your reach or they somehow compromise your recovery. Don't place unnecessary burdens on yourself, even though your intentions are admirable and your work ethic unassailable. Your brain injury is a bigger burden than most people can even imagine. Remember job number one: Recover from your brain injury. Don't put yourself in an environment or engage in activities that will set back your recovery. Recognize your limitations, and don't think you're a bad or lazy person because you don't volunteer for things like you used to.

The book sale

About nine months after my injury our town library prepared for its annual book sale. The call went out for volunteers to help sort through all of the donated books, tapes and CDs. I figured I had some free time because my recovery team had not approved my return to work, so I put my name down as available. One Saturday morning I showed up at the barn and another volunteer showed me what I would be doing: taking out books from boxes and setting them on tables set up at various parts of the barn: History, Environment, Fiction, Classics and so on.

After about 15 minutes of sorting and decision-making ("Is this a memoir or fiction?"), my brain started overheating. To use a different metaphor, it felt like my brain was one big bruise and I kept pushing on it. I knew I needed to stop, but out of embarrassment and stubbornness, I didn't just leave. Another job that needed doing was to stand outside the barn alone, taking each discarded box and either stamping on it or taking it apart by hand to flatten it, and toss the more-or-less flattened box onto a pile. I much preferred this solo activity, which I did for awhile and then went home to recover from the cognitive exertion.

Peer counseling

About two years into my injury I was recommended to be a part of a peer counseling group. Not knowing what to expect, I showed up at a meeting that was intended to train those interested in participating, about ten of us. I knew I was in trouble when I looked at the agenda. It was going to be a three-hour meeting. I knew I couldn't do anything for three hours. Rather than state this to the group, I decided to at least start and see how long I could hold on.

As we introduced ourselves, I found I was the only survivor in the group. All the others were family members of survivors. The facilitator started at the other end of the table and had people read short scenarios and role-play survivor and counselor. As the other participants tried their hand at this, I became increasingly overwhelmed. For one thing, professionally I used to write role-plays, and in much greater detail and complexity. Yet here I struggled following the simplest scenario, and I knew my turn was coming up.

I became more saturated with information as we continued around the table, and I felt my cognitive energies depleting just keeping track of their improvised responses in their roles. When my turn came, I was supposed to play a counselor and interact spontaneously with my partner, who played a truck driver with a TBI. As we began, my mind was blank. I didn't even know what to say, especially while all the other participants were watching me. I began to get choked up, and the facilitator came over to me and gently encouraged me to keep going. He said, "You can do this!" My mind still a blank, and my emotions getting the better of me, I said, "I'm telling you, I can't do this."

I went out of character and tried to level with him and the group about why this was so hard. I said something about the truck driver being in a wheelchair and one of the volunteers said, "You don't say 'in a wheelchair.' If a person uses a cane you don't say he is in a cane." I said, "Great, I can't even get the vernacular right."

Another volunteer, a father of a severely brain-injured man, said, "I think you should be a counselor. It will be good for you." I looked at him, but I kept silent. What I wanted to say was, "You know, people always think they know what brain-injury survivors should be doing. Trust me, I shouldn't be doing this. I understand reaching out and helping others but this is setting back my recovery." The meeting ended, I went home, and when I emerged from my dark room I e-mailed my regrets and said I would not be able to continue with the program.

So sometimes you have to stand up for yourself. Don't let someone who doesn't know your injury intimately make you feel like you should or shouldn't be doing a particular thing. You don't need to feel guilty on top of everything else you're going through.

So what did I learn?

Do I look back on those attempts at volunteering as defeats? No, I don't – though at the time, I felt pretty defeated and they weren't exactly victories either. They were just milestones marking the bumps along the way to recovery. Do what you can because there are a lot of needs out there, but trust what you know about your injury and the optimal environments for your recovery from your very individual brain injury. Don't measure your accomplishments next to another survivor's because every injury is different and every survivor's recovery is unique. We are all capable of many things but we are also capable of only so much.

MOVING ON TO MORE INTIMATE RELATIONSHIPS

We've seen how hard it can be to interact even with friends. Because family relationships tend to be more intense and complicated – more *important* – brain injury survivors often find it easier to spend time alone than risk alienating the people they love the most. This effort at self-preservation, this self-exile, has huge implications for the survivor's feelings of unraveling self-worth, loneliness, and creeping depression.

And the survivor's absence can, of course, further burden the family in all kinds of ways. We'll explore this in the next chapter.

21 – Spouses and Partners

HEATHER AND HER BOYFRIEND

"The dog and pony show"

Not long after Heather's brain injury (Chapter 9), her boyfriend spent the day rock climbing, something they had enjoyed together before her injury. She "wasn't having a great brain day," but she planned dinner for just the two of them and was looking forward to his return so she "wouldn't be lonely and could hear about his adventures":

> On his way back he called to tell me that he was bringing a few friends. I told him that I was having a pretty awful day. Could he reconsider? I told him that company might be a bad idea and suggested that they all go out for pizza instead. I couldn't think of a more polite or diplomatic alternative to what I was really thinking: I'm having an awful day; don't you dare bring people over. I actually pleaded with him the best way I knew how, but he seemed to think everything would be okay. My anxiety level was incredibly high because he still seemed to think that everything was going to be rainbows.
>
> So I made dinner for everyone and then hid in my bedroom, crying like mad. [My boyfriend] brought dinner to my bedside and asked me why I couldn't come down. The only thing I could manage to say was that I just couldn't do it. I imagine that it was pretty hard for him to understand. Plus, I get worse when someone presses me to explain why I feel I can't do whatever it is that I'm having anxiety about doing. And that intensifies the anxiety.

Like any brain-injured person, Heather doesn't want people to see her when she is in the middle of a meltdown, and it is especially upsetting in front of a loved one. "The worst part" is that her boyfriend sees her in her "worst states."

He also sees her come out of a bad meltdown and try her best "to be sugar and sunshine" for family and friend get-togethers. She knows that he wonders about the shift in what looks like her moods, a phenomenon that Heather refers to as her "dog and pony show":

> It's to make other people feel comfortable around me, but it's hard for me to accomplish cognitively. I worry about saying the wrong thing. I smile a lot and try to ladle out compliments to people. I try to be involved in conversations, but feel the wear and tear on my brain. When no one is listening, I tell [my boyfriend] that I can't think of words, and that I'm having trouble. I walk outside and stare at clouds. After the event, I have "cognitive hangover."

Heather confided her biggest fear. Her boyfriend might end their relationship "to find a girl who isn't brain-injured." Many brain-injured people suffer similar insecurities.

VANESSA AND CLIVE

"Damaged goods"

Vanessa and Clive are not their real names, but they *are* English. Vanessa, like Heather, contacted me after seeing "You Look Great!" and we have been friends and confidants ever since. We try to offer each other support and encouragement, and this mutual reaching out has helped us both.

Vanessa recently told me she was getting married, and confided that her brain injury was creating difficulties for her and her fiancé, Clive:

> Things are already going to be a struggle with this engagement. I have problems that I deal with everyday and to be honest I am sad at the moment when I should be happy. Clive's brother is causing a big

> problem in our relationship. I don't know if I have the strength to deal with the issues that his brother and his family are causing.

We e-mailed a little about this, and we agreed that it's better not to be married than to be married to the wrong person. It emerged though that Clive may well be the right person and that it is his brother who is poisoning things, not because his brother is hard-hearted, but because he doesn't understand the effects of the injury:

> Clive had a talk with his brother. One thing that has hit me hard and I'm having a difficult time not thinking about is, he asked, "When is Vanessa going back to work?"
>
> When I spent time with Clive's family his brother noticed that I took longer than most people to get going during the day when I was there and said, "Vanessa may be sick." Well, he doesn't know about my problems but Clive does. Clive told me, "It's none of his business when you go back to work."
>
> I have thought that I would like to try and go back to prove myself but I am not able to at this time. I don't know when I will be. Clive loves me no matter what the circumstances and wants to be with me but I AM NOTHING BUT DAMAGED GOODS IF THEY FIND OUT ABOUT ME AND MY PROBLEMS.

I hear this term "damaged goods" from other survivors in a variety of contexts; the phrase is tinged with pain and longing for our brains and our lives to be the way they once were.

TBI: A MAJOR CRISIS FOR ANY RELATIONSHIP

I waited about six months before I went to my first TBI support group. I was not prepared for how it would affect me. Two of the guys I talked with, both about eight years into their injury, told me all about their painful divorces. One man, driving with his wife, three kids, and a niece, had a moose walk in front of the car. His wife stuck by him through some really bad times at first, but at some point it all became too much for her.

The other survivor I talked with, a lawyer, had had a brain tumor and his wife stuck by him for seven years. They too were in the process of a divorce made especially painful because of their three kids.

I left absolutely depleted and depressed. The stories I listened to were so disheartening (divorce!) and discouraging (eight years of injury!) that I avoided the group for over a year. I refused to allow myself to imagine even the possibility that my injury would affect my marriage. Nevertheless, as Gregg's wife Diana observes, "TBI is a major crisis for even the strongest marriage."

GREGG AND DIANA

"TBI changes your whole perception of self, reality, and the world, and everything is different for him. That's hard for us to understand." Diana

Gregg not the life of the party anymore

Gregg's injury (Chapter 2) became a crisis for his wife Diana, but she says she stepped up and dealt with it as she would any crisis in her life. Her biggest loss was Gregg's former vivacity and sociability:

> Gregg was always the life of the party. He was very funny and loved
> to create fun and chaotic family events – big parties, funky
> decorations, feasts of food. I remember one time he hid appetizers all
> over the house, and for my 40th birthday he put on a big cookout in the
> yard and hid all kinds of stuffed animals in the yard for the kids to
> discover. He was always the catalyst for a lot of laughs. Gregg was
> always the party guy.

Gregg cannot handle parties anymore, and that's been a big adjustment for them both. Diana has so much anxiety about the family's annual Christmas Eve party, a big event they used to enjoy together, that when Gregg began to participate in them again she decided to schedule chores for herself. "This way I don't have to see him suffer through it. I'd just as soon not see him suffering."

Diana says that Gregg has made a lot of progress in many areas, but "no progress in the party department, except that he figured out it helped to go early and stay briefly."

No more pig piles

The injury affected their family life in other ways. They always enjoyed having all their grandchildren over at the same time ("Gregg loved pig piles"), but because the noise and chaos exact a terrible toll on him, they have had to adapt by having their grandchildren over one at a time. She misses the "grandchildren fests."

Protecting the marriage relationship

"Gregg says there's not a moment when he doesn't know he's changed," Diana adds. "TBI changes your whole perception of self, reality, and the world, and everything is different for him. That's hard for us to understand." Despite the tumultuous changes, Diana says that they have figured out how to protect their own relationship.

For roughly two years, their relationship shrank to the dimensions of Gregg's injury. It was all they thought and talked about, although "for the first three or four months there was absolutely no conversation; Gregg was feeling too miserable." Although the injury dominated their lives, as time passed and Gregg made progress in therapy and in groups focused on family support strategies, their conversation became "a bit more natural." Diana reports that "now there are plenty of times when [the injury] is not always the center of conversation."

Diana explains that Gregg works very hard to maintain a good relationship with her and "makes an effort to be there" for her when she needs to talk about her own problems. But what makes TBI so hard on a marriage is that the survivor is so often "in a state of flux":

> Emotions for both of us range from really hopeful to terrible anxiety. I'm happy when he's having a good day and I despair, as he does, when he's having a bad day. I know I'm not isolated yet sometimes it's hard not to feel isolated when I need emotional support and he's just not capable of providing it in a moment when I need it.
>
> I also have this hyper-awareness and hyper-vigilance. We might be watching something funny on TV and I'll laugh out loud, and he winces because it hurts him and it's painful. I have to always be a little on guard about how he's feeling and then control my own responses. It's not like I'm walking on ice or on tiptoe, but I can't be completely spontaneous and natural because I have to be so tuned in to how Gregg is feeling.

She says that Gregg is worth all the challenges. "My marriage is still very good. It's just different. The essence of Gregg is still there. He's still the essential Gregg I fell in love with."

TOM AND ARTHUR

Tom and Arthur (Chapter 2) had been in a domestic partnership for four years at the time of Tom's car wreck. As often happens in the first weeks after an accident, they focused so intently on Tom's physical injuries – his crushed nerve in his neck – that neither thought about the possibility that Tom's brain might have been injured. Arthur recalls that a few weeks after Tom's accident "the anxiety came":

> I'm a licensed independent clinical social worker with 30 years of mental- health treatment experience and I could see that Tom's anxiety was off the charts. First it was the night sweats to the point where the sheets and bed coverings were soaked. Then the panic attacks came. He had a debilitating loss of breath, intense fear of loss of consciousness, and such overwhelming anxiety that he was completely incapacitated.
>
> He was also having nightmares about the accident every night. He'd wake up screaming in his sleep – often he'd be calling out to the other driver – and he'd wake up sobbing.

Arthur had extensive experience working with clients who suffered from anxiety disorders, but he still felt unprepared for living with someone as the symptoms manifested:

> Tom had an overwhelming fearfulness of people and situations and couldn't even walk into a grocery store. He was a shell of himself. He would curl up in a ball in a corner upstairs. He couldn't take himself to

> see the psychiatrist across the street – I had to ask his mother to go
> with him.

Arthur had replaced the wrecked car with an earlier model of the exact same car, but Tom's anxiety was so great that he refused to get into it. He would not leave the house. Then Tom became manic, he cried easily for no apparent reason, and could not concentrate or sleep.

As I mentioned in an earlier chapter, Tom's employer stuck to the position that his difficulties were unrelated to the accident. Ultimately Tom lost his job and all his benefits.

The psychic and monetary cost

Arthur says that among the most difficult challenges he and Tom had to face was the refusal of attorneys, doctors, the bank's insurance company, and the worker's comp administration to recognize that the injury he sustained in the car accident was the cause of Tom's problems:

> Everyone involved felt that Tom's physical problems were legitimate,
> but we spent almost two years defending him against accusations that
> his symptoms were the result of a pre-existing condition. [The
> insurance company's] psychiatrist interviewed him for one hour and
> concluded that they were caused by Tom having closeted his
> homosexuality!

Outraged, Tom and Arthur went to court. The court-appointed psychiatrist concluded that Tom's symptoms were not a pre-existing condition, thereby overruling the insurance company, but the judge and their lawyer – they actually used several lawyers and are still paying legal bills out of pocket – warned that the only way to settle quickly was to agree to eliminate the "psychiatric" component from their case. Otherwise they would face an additional three to five more years of fighting.

They had spent almost two years battling the insurance company's judgment that Tom's condition was "pre-existing." The thought of another grueling five years of struggle so demoralized them, and the prospect of the financial costs so overwhelmed them, that they agreed. But it pained them to retreat from proving that Tom's symptoms were caused by the injury, and the aspersions that the insurance company, the bank, and the bank's Human Resources Center cast on their integrity "still bother us today." Arthur adds:

> To be candid, the hardest part was that so few people believed our day-to-day reality. To this day that still makes me sad. The last thing we tried to do is rob the system. We just wanted to be treated the way we should have been. Tom's disability genuinely affected his day-to-day life – and ours as a couple. Because we were partnered and not married, we couldn't get any benefits so I paid for every psychiatric intervention out of pocket – everything. We had to make decisions about buying food or medication.
>
> Case workers would come to our home and see that it was nice and deny benefits partially because we had a nice place, and because they concluded that Tom wasn't "severe" and "persistently" mentally ill, nor did he fit the description of what's referred to in the mental health profession as the "worried well." So he fell through the cracks of the Department of Mental Health. He fell through the cracks of a broken system.

Before continuing with Tom and Arthur's story, I must emphasize two points:

- Lingering sensations of sadness and even bitterness at shabby treatment are common among survivors.

- TBI survivors often hear remarks from professionals – whether medical, legal, or insurance – that diminish the injury and discount suffering. We must be firm about how the injury has affected every area of our lives, and persist in legal matters or unemployment and disability issues, even though they can leave us feeling demoralized and demeaned.

"The injury affects every aspect of our lives"

Before Tom's accident, the couple had a lot of friends and a rich, full social life. Today, they mostly confine themselves to their home where Tom spends a lot of "therapy time" sitting quietly on a stone bench in the lovely, pine-shaded garden outside their living-room doors.

Tom's injured brain has completely changed both of their lives. It determines the way they schedule their time, the people they can be with, and the settings they can manage – and they always have an exit strategy in any situation that requires social interaction. Arthur says that "reading where Tom's anxiety is" has become as much a part of their lives as other daily tasks.

They have to plan even family events. When Arthur's daughter graduated from Boston University, Arthur knew that Tom would be unable to negotiate the trip and the ceremony unless he carefully choreographed the day. To avoid a long car trip, which Tom still finds excruciating, the two took the train into Boston. At the graduation ceremony they sat in the back so Tom could leave easily, and they passed up the celebratory dinner in the graduate's honor.

Public places continue to be a huge challenge for Tom. He used to do his sales work in bank offices in supermarkets, but for months after the accident he could not set foot inside a grocery "with all those people." Arthur worked with him so that "we increased his exposure to the supermarket in little bits."

So the challenges remain, but Tom and Arthur feel that they have "weathered the storms and come through them." Arthur likes to say, "We're battered, but we're not beaten."

These stories of Heather and her boyfriend, Vanessa and Clive, Gregg and Diana, Tom and Arthur present some common themes, such as the need for both partners to communicate clearly, be patient, show empathy, and be willing to sacrifice on behalf of the other. These stories illustrate how, even though specific brain injuries vary widely in their sequelae, many of the same coping strategies help when trying to nurture and strengthen a relationship. That is the subject of the next chapter.

22 – Tips and Strategies for Couples

TIPS AND SURVIVOR ANECDOTES

What follows are some tips that can help any of us in a relationship, and anecdotes I have collected from fellow survivors that helped me create the tips.

Tip 1:

TBI requires that couples take extra pains to communicate very clearly to prevent bad feelings from festering. Spouses and partners of a TBI survivor need to remember that TBI is a disability, and survivors need to keep in mind how severely the injury can affect the lives of loved ones.

Survivor anecdote: The "Hose Incident"

Those of you who are familiar with the comic strip Calvin & Hobbes will remember the alluded to but never revealed "spaghetti incident." For those of you who haven't read Calvin & Hobbes, all you need to know is that the incident must have been such a horror show that Calvin's mother and father never talked about it. They would just shudder at the memory.

Well, Bill says he sort of shudders about "the hose incident" but he told me about it anyway.

"Saturday is chore day in our house. We make a run to the dump, do yard work, and whatever else is on our list. Nobody in the family just sits around idle on Saturday until the chores are done. And something usually needs doing on our farm."

This particular Saturday morning Bill's wife Amy was up unusually early, and she started putting new fabric on the couch in their bedroom. He got up shortly thereafter, and because he'd already made the dump run on Wednesday, he sat down at his electric keyboard to play a little new music. He was learning the rudiments of reading music and decided to try to transcribe what he was playing onto blank sheet music. He found this great fun and it felt therapeutic to him.

About 45 minutes later Bill saw Amy through the front door hauling two heavy hoses across their front deck, and she looked annoyed. Bill thought, "Uh oh . . ." Despite his diminished ability to read body language and facial expressions – not long after his injury Amy told him quite bluntly that he couldn't decipher nonverbal signals, including hers – after 25 years of marriage, he knew that look. Bill had thought Amy was upstairs putting fabric on the couch and all of a sudden she materialized on their deck – and she was not happy.

He put the keyboard down, jumped out of his chair, and hustled out the front door. "Let me take those from you!"

"No!"

"Why are you angry?"

"I'm not angry!"

"Is it because I'm playing the piano?"

"No!"

He kept asking what was on her mind, and then Amy started to cry. She hardly ever cries. She finally said, "I feel like there's so much to do and if I don't do it, it won't get done. And I'm concerned that it's 9:45, and if you don't do the things on your list now, you won't do them at all."

What she said was honest and accurate. Amy often leaves a short list for Bill and each of their children on the counter. She knew that when Bill hits a cognitive wall he has to retreat to the back bedroom to recover. If he gets busy doing other things and doesn't get the chores done early in the day, they either don't get done or Amy ends up having to do them herself.

You know how every once in a while you say the right thing? This hardly ever happens. The French even have a term for thinking of the right thing to say after it's too late: *esprit d'escalier*; literally, "staircase wit," because you think of it after you've left the room. Bill thinks that on this day he actually said the right thing. He said, "Amy, you need to tell me what you are thinking. With this injury I don't read situations so well, and I don't always read you so well."

Bill finds it hard to read facial expressions and body language – it's all he can do to figure what his own brain is telling him to do – so his limitations in this area have created new challenges for them as a couple.

He continued, "I need you to communicate really openly with me. You could have opened the front door and said, 'I need help.' I thought you were upstairs working on your project and I figured that we had the rest of the day to do all our chores." He convinced Amy to let him handle the hoses, which he bundled up separately, strapped with bungee cords, and hauled to the basement.

Tip 2:

Always be sensitive to the enormous strain your spouse is under because of your injury.

Survivor anecdote

> I groaned thinking of going to a Christmas party with our closest friends. I knew it would be an abrasive environment for my head. My wife had a great idea: go about an hour after it started because the first hour was just standing around talking with drinks anyway. So I showed up a little late, and it was great way to pace myself for the rest of evening.

Survivor anecdote

> In the first year of my injury, a car hit our beloved cat in front of our house. A neighbor carried him up to us as we stood on our front porch. My wife cried on and off all day. I asked her later, "Why did it hit you so hard?" and she said, "I think because if I cried for you I would never stop."

Tip 3:

Both spouses must go out of their way to hold out a hand, to hug and show affection, to say "I love you." These might sound easy and even cliché, but if you feel undesirable your sense of self-worth can go right down the toilet. Depression is about two minutes away.

Survivor anecdote

> By far the hardest part of this injury has been the persistent and stultifying feeling that my injury has somehow made my very presence an imposition. Because of my crushed feelings of self-worth and attractiveness, there's a deep rift in my marriage and my husband isn't

even aware of it. Because I feel so undesired and undesirable to him I often go to bed broken-hearted. I told him that this is my greatest suffering, not the injury itself.

When someone commits suicide people always say, "Why didn't she say something?" I'm not there yet but I told him how unhappy I am, how sad, and how my feelings are really hurt and that I need his love and affection.

Tip 4:

Sometimes what you think is a selfless choice can hurt others. Resist your urges to be heroic and do more than you should because the cognitive fatigue that results is likely to cost your family members.

Survivor anecdote

I had an hour lunch with a friend and called home to say I would stop and pick up some groceries afterwards. My husband urged me to resist my compulsion to help out given I'd just expended a ton of cognitive energy over lunch, but I did anyway. I agreed afterwards this was a big mistake to ignore his advice because I had to retreat from the family for the rest of the day.

Tip 5:

If she does something that flummoxes you, explain your dilemma. Your new life will be full of moments like this. Stay calm, and try to explain from your perspective what just happened.

Survivor anecdote

My son and I agreed we'd have dinner at the pancake house, buy him some new sneakers, and then try out a new gym together. I had thought through the geography and the timing of this, and felt good about it. At the moment my wife walked into the room, I was thinking about something else. This meant that I had to switch gears – always a tricky cognitive maneuver – to tell her our plan. She innocently suggested that we reverse the order of the itinerary.

I looked at her and didn't know what to say so I started stammering. She said, "It was just a suggestion!" and walked away. I won't try and deconstruct the multiple layers of that interaction, but I tried – slowly, painfully – to explain my dilemma . . . that I didn't have a negative feeling about her suggestion; I was just trying to process it.

Tip 6:

Your spouse should expect to sort through another layer of complexity and stress at social functions. Remind yourselves that, as hard as it is sometimes, it's still important for you to see your friends.

Survivor anecdote

My husband is great when it comes to looking out for me in social settings. I have seen him ask the hostess to turn the music way down, or he might see me having a difficult conversation with someone and, like at a high school dance, cut in and take it from there.

Spouse anecdote

Sometimes I'll walk into a crowded room and right away I'll think, "Oh no, this isn't good for her." Even if the occasion is fun for me, it is less so because I know it will be hard on her. We agree that it's important for us as a couple to socialize, but during a party I often find myself fretting about her well-being. We figured out that it's okay for her to leave early, or to remove herself to another room for awhile.

Tip 7:

Messy piles of stuff cause cognitive indigestion for everyone in your household. They are unhealthy to look at, and embarrassing when people visit. When you make your to-do list for the day, put "clean up one mess" at the top. By the end of one week, if all goes according to plan, which is subject to change based on how you are feeling, you will have cleaned up seven messes.

Survivor anecdote

> One of my wife's biggest stressors is seeing messy piles of miscellaneous papers and clothing around the house. Organizing messy piles of same is often one of the hardest things a TBI survivor has to do. It's not that we don't see the messes, but we see so many categories of things – bills, letters, articles torn out to read later – that we have a hard time figuring what to do first and where everything goes.
>
> I started putting stuff I didn't know where to put into my car. It didn't take long for my car to look like it belonged to a crazy person. I realized if I picked up our daughter and one of her friends I would have to shove everything over to one side. Eventually I was sufficiently humiliated to attack the mess and put everything away. I felt about 100 pounds lighter and less obviously brain-injured.

Tip 8:

If you go away on vacation together, encourage your spouse to go have fun whenever you need to recharge your battery.

Survivor anecdote

> When we visited San Francisco, my wife and I took a long walk through the city and across the Golden Gate Bridge. It was a gorgeous day, and she wanted to keep walking. I was ready to head back to the

hotel in a taxi, which she totally understood. After my two-hour nap, we met for dinner, both feeling refreshed.

Tip 9:

Ask "permission" to complain. This gives you freedom to say what's really on your mind without making complaints a normal part of your conversation. You can also say, "Can you just come over here and hold my hand?"

Survivor anecdote

> One day I was feeling especially bad, but I didn't want to just launch into it when my husband walked into the room. This injury dominates the survivor's life in so many ways, and we keep so much to ourselves because we don't want to harp on it. It also must be taxing or at least boring to listen to all the time. I also didn't want to add to his burdens just then, but I wanted to be honest with him.
>
> I took a different tack. Knowing he would say yes, I asked him, "Can I complain?" He said sure, so I said, "I feel terrible and my ears have never rung louder than right now." It made me feel better just to say that.

Tip 10:

We'd rather it be said about us that we act heroically every day than "he gets tired easily."

Survivor anecdote

> Early in the injury I overheard my wife on the phone answering a relative's questions about me, and it irritated me to hear, "He sleeps a lot," and "He gets tired easily." While this was true, I spoke to her and likened the injury to that of Boston Celtics star Kevin McHale who in 1987 played the finals against the Lakers on a broken foot. Watching

him you would not have guessed he had a broken foot; he played ferociously and now we know heroically.

Tip 11:

Make every effort to be engaging on topics other than TBI!

Survivor anecdote

Living day to day with your brain injury is all-consuming because it's the filter through which you now see everything. To your spouse your preoccupation with brain injury can begin to feel like the "other woman." She might get demoralized if you show more energy and are more engaged when your conversation relates to brain injury generally, whether your own or that of others.

STRATEGIES FOR COUPLES

The following pages consolidate a lot of great advice from fellow survivors and their spouses or partners. I have organized the information by these themes:

- Conflict Management
- Anger Management
- Despair Management
- Nurture Management

- Family Management
- Relationship Management
- Logistics Management
- Injury Management

Most of the strategies can apply to both partners, injured and not. Strategies specifically for either spouse should be apparent.

Conflict Management

Strategy	Examples or Tactics
Think before you speak	If you feel that you can't discuss an issue rationally, stop and walk away. Tell your partner that you are taking a breather so you can refocus. You're not walking away from the problem; you're just taking a few minutes to reconsider what you really want to say.
Double your efforts to communicate openly and honestly	<ul><li>Survivors can be ultra-sensitive to oblique criticisms of their behavior. For example, if you say "buck up" or "do more" survivors are likely to think that you don't understand their challenges.</li><li>Survivors are also likely to despair at the implication that there is nothing seriously wrong with them, and this may cause withdrawal out of frustration and resentment that they have to use slender reserves of emotional and mental energy to "prove" it to you.</li></ul>
Sometimes you need to just listen, without interjecting your own thoughts	<ul><li>Obviously, you can't know what's on your partner's mind without listening.</li><li>Your partner probably doesn't want you to offer advice ("You should do this; you shouldn't do that") or to act as a therapist.</li><li>Just listen attentively – without interrupting or dispensing judgment – so your partner is confident that you are giving your full attention to what is being said, even if you don't agree or even fully understand.</li></ul>

Notes:

Anger Management

Strategy	Examples or Tactics
Give yourself permission to be angry, but be sure to work through it so you can move on	• Having a brain injury or living with someone with a brain injury can produce a lot of anger, but you have to learn to express it constructively. • If you get mad, express it in appropriate ways, but don't deny your own feelings as a way to protect your partner. Be as honest and upfront as possible.
Learn healthy ways to express anger	• Anger is a valid feeling, but you have to work together to find ways to express it appropriately. That will help to protect your relationship. • Avoid making statements in an accusative tone such as, "What were you thinking?" Instead say, "It's not you I'm angry at; I'm angry at the injury." • Be careful with your body language. For example, don't sigh heavily or roll your eyes. That kind of thing shouts your disapproval and frustration. Instead ask, "How can I help or make this situation better?" or "Help me think through the challenge of the moment."
Learn how to quarrel differently	• Survivors often have to remove themselves if a disagreement escalates. They need more time to process information and emotion so couples take longer to come to agreements. But the wait is worth it for the resolution. • Don't walk on eggshells, worried that your partner will crack.

Anger Management, cont'd.

Strategy	Examples or Tactics
Be angry at the condition, not at your partner	• Absolve your partner from the discomfort this condition caused you, no matter how personally you might be inclined to interpret the situation. • For example, "I recognize that you are not trying to make things more difficult for me or that you are deliberately being resistant. I don't take the manifestations of your sequelae personally. You don't get to choose when your brain chemistry changes."

Notes:

Despair Management

Strategy	Examples or Tactics
Anticipate feelings of despair, but act to work through it	Stay tuned to your emotional state. Try to recognize anxiety and/or depressive symptoms and see a professional if you have ongoing concerns.
Realize that some good thing might come out of your injury	"An injured partner changes your life, but you can adapt and find life good. Arthur is putting his experience with me to good use. He now has a large number of clients with anxiety disorders." *(Tom)*
Clearly define success	<ul><li>Anticipate that your expectations of each other might be too high.</li><li>"Arthur generally feels that I should be doing more and he expects more out of me. For example, he wants me to get back in the car and drive, and that's too hard." *(Tom)*</li></ul>
Assure each other that you might eventually have an even better, more fulfilling life than before the injury but it will take time	Survivors want their injury to go away so that they can have their old lives back. While that might be unattainable, they need your assurance that together you can get through the toughest times on the way to building a new life together.
Be careful not to raise the bar of expectations too high	<ul><li>Sometimes when your non-injured partner sees you do something that is a big step forward, they think you can do it every time. This raises the bar. Instead, your partner should allow you to raise your own expectations. Otherwise your non-injured partner is pushing expectations and setting you up to fail.</li><li>Be encouraging through every struggle, regardless of past performance.</li></ul>

Despair Management, cont'd

Strategy	Examples or Tactics
Expect to feel isolated, so orchestrate times for socializing	• TBI forces couples to work together to address a lot of issues. When you have a child with an issue it's stressful, but it can also unite couples. Both you and your spouse have to deal with the injury – and all the little logistics and decisions and fallouts that cascade from it. • As a couple you are addressing TBI from two different perspectives, ones that can isolate you from each other. Work at building empathy in each other by appropriately communicating what you're going through.
Don't let anyone else define your reality for you	"People would tell me that Tom and I seemed fine and that the after-effects of the accident were gone. They did not and could not know or understand our reality." *(Arthur)*

Notes:

Nurture Management

Strategy	Examples or Tactics
Ask for help when you need it	"Gregg is not one to ask for help and can be pretty stubborn, but asking for my help can help prevent or at least minimize the cognitive hangovers that are so hard on us both. I'm happy to go to the store or take over cooking the dinner if it will salvage an evening for us." *(Diana)*
Be sensitive that survivors often have self-esteem issues	• Help your injured partner continue to build confidence by saying things such as, "You can do this. Don't give up. Maybe it will take you longer, but you can do this." • Offer to discuss a task before your injured partner attempts to complete it. Say, "Let's talk about it first. Let's make a plan." That can help build the "I can do" feeling because it makes them think first and increases the likelihood of success. Success will make that task easier to do the second time. • "If you were an active functional individual who was independent and successful, the injury can take it all away in a minute. Your self-esteem is injured every time you are forced to recognize a new limitation you didn't know existed." *(Arthur)*
Continually encourage your partner	• Survivors need to be told that their partner believes in them, and has a lot of confidence in them. • If the injured spouse does fail, give ample assurance that you don't define him or her by that failure and still believe that success is possible.
Be consoling	"When Arthur comes home from work and sees me in the garden he will ask me, 'Are you okay?' Simple kindnesses and expressions of concern soothe, reassure, and cheer your injured partner." *(Tom)*

Nurture Management, cont'd

Strategy	Examples or Tactics
Be gentle and understanding about why he might be pushing himself too hard	Survivors try to do too much because they: • Know you are overburdened and have to take on so much extra work all the time • Are trying to compensate for their inability to work and earn their former income • Hope the effort might help regain self-respect • Can't recognize their over-exertion point • Push themselves to do more on good days • Want to have a semblance of a normal life
When your injured spouse is in "crash" mode, touch is very important	Due to noise and chaos, survivors crave solitude, yet in solitude get lonely. Check in once in a while. You don't have to say anything, but they will appreciate your touch. Squeeze a hand gently or stroke their back.
When people ask how the survivor is doing, choose language that emphasizes the positive instead of the negative	• E.g., "He never gives up," "She is incredibly determined," "I'm so proud of him," "She has come a long way, and she's got a long road ahead of her." • Avoid saying things like, "He wears down easily." This rankles because it fails to suggest the progress survivors have made, or how heroic they are just getting through the day. • If they have been hitting the gym as part of their rehab, say that they're getting in great shape physically.

Nurture Management, cont'd

Strategy	Examples or Tactics
Identify a trusted person who is a good listener and willing to listen to you regularly	• Support groups aren't for everybody, but at one time or another everybody needs support. Even if you are a private person, sharing with a friend can alleviate many stresses. • Try an online support group (e.g., dailystrength.com). • Agree that you will listen to your "Listening Partner" in return for the favor.

Notes:

Family Management

Strategy	Examples or Tactics
Family members should be forthright about communicating their thoughts and feelings, even if they prefer not to because of their protective feelings for the survivor	• TBI has diminished survivors' ability to read people and situations, including their closest family members. • "I've learned to communicate my feelings to him directly, even if I'm inclined to avoid burdening him." *(Lynne)*
For the family's sake, be brave enough to try to do some of the things you did together before the injury	• If you celebrated holidays with family members before the injury and you're both wary of celebrating them the same way, do them differently. • Celebrate holidays more quietly, perhaps on a different day. It's important to have a happy time; it doesn't matter when it is. Come up with celebrations and traditions that work for you and your family.
Be as involved as the survivor wants you to be in meetings with members of her recovery team	• Meet with your injured spouse's licensed social worker and be aware that the social worker might direct many questions to you. • It's important to have a time and place to talk about family issues that might not be raised otherwise. A skillful social worker can orchestrate a discussion that can be fruitful for everybody. It's healthy for family members to air their feelings. • Include one or more of your children in the meeting because your social worker can evaluate how they seem to be coping with the effects of the injury on the family and make valuable suggestions.

Notes:

Relationship Management

Strategy	Examples or Tactics
Acknowledge that TBI is like a mistress who has gone nuts, like Glenn Close in "Fatal Attraction."	"This sounds very negative, but your injured spouse does not adore TBI; he is enslaved to it. It takes most of his thoughts, energy, and interest. I know that I am important and much loved and adored, but I am second to this injury. This has to be true of every TBI marriage." *(Lynne)*
Anticipate frustration and prepare ahead of time how to deal with it	"The most frustrating thing for us was that people refused to believe that Tom's accident caused a head trauma which was followed by PTSD symptoms. That traumatized him and me again and again." *(Arthur)*
Be flexible and adapt to your new life together	"Life will be different because of having to adjust to where you go, who you are with, and whether or not the environment you're in will work. You have to make changes because of the injury, so try to adapt and be patient." *(Arthur)*
Be creative about getting your emotional and social needs met	<ul><li>Although your spouse is likely to be supportive, she might not be the best person to depend on.</li><li>Take time away from your partner occasionally. For example, make an effort to continue enjoying your hobbies and interests.</li><li>Meet other family members who face similar challenges, and share strategies and tactics.</li><li>"I would lose myself completely in the struggle to help Tom if I failed to regularly schedule down time for myself." *(Arthur)*</li></ul>

Relationship Management, cont'd

Strategy	Examples or Tactics
Consider seeing a psychotherapist or attend a support group, individually or together	• Psychotherapy – whether a neuropsychiatrist or neuropsychologist – can dedicate time to check in with your needs inventory and address your issues. • You might find it very helpful to talk with people who understood what you are both going through.
Expect the role of caregiver to expand	TBI makes the partner part advisor, sympathizer, mother (or father), nag, observer, "suggester" – and these all exist in any marriage already. TBI intensifies and amplifies these roles.
When you are both up for it, take time to listen to each other's problems, stories, and complaints	"This is the biggest thing for me. There are many times when Gregg is incapable of interaction and the spontaneous things don't happen. This hurts. I know that this is due to the physical injury, but sometimes it feels like an emotional wall." *(Diana)*
Plan time together for fun a couple of times a month	• Commit to an uncomplaining flexibility if you have to cancel and reschedule. • "We have to cancel our plans and reschedule all the time because rainy and even cloudy days almost always intensify his difficulties. Since we live in New England where the weather is notoriously unpredictable, I have learned to adapt." *(Diana)* • Feel free to go out by yourself if, for example, you've bought tickets to a show and your partner can't make it. • "Every Sunday at 5:00 we turn off our cell phones and computers and shut off the outside world completely. It's a time for us to tune in to one another and make plans for the coming week." *(Arthur)*

Relationship Management, cont'd

Strategy	Examples or Tactics
Avoid talking about the effects of the injury 24/7	Make an agreement to avoid talk about the injury for a few hours or days. This will ultimately make your time together more interesting, and you will feel less dominated by the injury.

Notes:

Logistics Management

Strategy	Examples or Tactics
If at all possible, avoid traveling for extended periods that separate you from an especially needy partner	"I had been traveling nationally as a consultant when Tom was in the early stages of his injury and his symptoms completely overwhelmed him. I was in Michigan giving a deposition and he was in a state – flipping out on the other end of the phone – and I had to get on a plane and come home. Now I do 75 percent clinical instead of consulting. I gave up all the traveling, the money, the great job, to stay close to home. Ultimately that made life a lot easier for both of us." *(Arthur)*
Anticipate a "danger zone" and retreat	• Follow through when your partner tells you to rest or retreat from a given situation. Your partner can often see that you're getting fatigued before you realize it. • "Since the injury I have learned to read him so well that I can tell by the expression in his eyes when he needs to remove himself from a situation. Sometimes though, out of his desire to be an attentive and loving husband, he fails to protect himself. The reason retreat is so important is that when he pushes himself 'until he gets the job done,' he gets to feeling so terrible that he can be sick for days, and I suffer along with him. It costs us both." *(Diana)*
Simplify! Rid yourself of as much stuff as you can and make up your mind to purchase less stuff.	• Clutter makes life even harder for a TBI survivor – and for the partner who may have to take over a lot of the housework. Stuff accumulating around the house makes messes that exhaust everybody, not just physically but psychically. • Minimizing the stuff you have to look at and think about will lighten the load for you and your whole family and will make you feel better.
Look at the coming week and plan accordingly	Try to anticipate any settings that might be problematic and look at a range of alternatives and back-up plans.

Logistics Management, cont'd

Strategy	Examples or Tactics
Run interference and anticipate what the injured partner can't	• Recognize that you might feel that you have to shelter your spouse from family problems and challenges, but keep in mind that any protective walls you build can create other challenges. The same walls that you build to protect your spouse can separate you from each other. • Consider your spouse's plans for the day or the week, and if you think he's planning to do too much, say so. You can see the big picture with greater clarity than the survivor can, so gently point out any events that could be eliminated or postponed. This might help prevent or at least minimize the possibility of a "crash" that affects the whole family as well as the survivor. • It's very helpful to say to a brain-injured person, "Slow it down. Take it down a notch. There's no hurry. Don't rush." It takes us longer to figure things out, and at the same time, we are anxious to complete a task, which makes us move faster and make mistakes. Encourage us to slow down and think. That way we can get it done the right way instead of having to do it a second time.
When it comes to presenting your case – whether with an insurance company, an employer or Social Security – be persistent; don't give up	"From the beginning we were turned down and turned away from a host of state and federal resources that were supposed to protect Americans with disabilities. Although Tom's former employer committed one egregious act of discrimination after another, and bullied us with their attorneys, we didn't give up our battle to be treated fairly and for the bank to accommodate us reasonably. When the bank through their Worker's Compensation attorney made false accusations against us and rejected our appeals repeatedly we did not give up." *(Arthur)*

Notes:

Injury Management

Strategy	Examples or Tactics
Give the survivor time to consider ideas and suggestions	• If a survivor fails to respond the moment you make a suggestion, it's because we are processing it, not necessarily because we are rejecting it. Be patient. Give us time to sort it out.
Try to avoid "energy leaks"	• Prioritizing can be hard for survivors, who can unwittingly spend time on things or people that are fun, but come at the expense of more important things. Family members should not get less of the injured person's limited attention. • Before you commit to an activity, ask yourself, "Should I do this – even if it's fun – or save my energy for family members?"
Come up with a word that your spouse can use to signal you that it's time for you to rest in a quiet room	• A simple signal can help to prevent or minimize a survivor's cognitive hangover, and benefits both partners. • Using one word is good because it eliminates discussion, and in social situations that protects our privacy. Whisper your word and your partner will know that it means to go rest now.
Allow and even encourage your partner plenty of time to be alone	• Your injured partner is not rejecting you when wanting "alone time," and sometimes survivors need isolation in large doses. • "I will sit in my garden for hours at a time and Arthur knows it is good medicine for me." *(Tom)*

Notes:

23 – Strategies for Children of the Injured

"GREAT, CHRIS MADE ANDREW A SHIRT!"

I lost certain basic coping skills and the ability to discern how to react to some things, especially surprises. I'll give you a "for instance." Our eldest son Chris was home from college, we hadn't seen him in awhile and it was great to have him back. It helps to know that Chris has a, shall we say, unique sense of humor: ironic, dark, you might even say post-modern. We get along very well; we like a lot of the same movies and laugh at a lot of the same things.

Lynne told me that Chris was up in his room making matching t-shirts for himself and our middle son Andrew, and I thought to myself, "That's nice!" Still marveling at this burst of fraternal generosity, I heard Chris open his door and down he bounded wearing his new t-shirt and holding Andrew's aloft, looking triumphant.

The large orange letters on the white t-shirts said: "GO 2 HELL!" Chris asked me, "Do you like it?" I just stood there, looking at him and his shirt. Even though I can be as post-modern as the next guy, I had no idea how to respond.

Think of how many things were going through my brain-injured head. I thought of him wearing it outside the house. I thought of Andrew wearing his outside the house. I thought of people, good and hard-working people, seeing my sons' "go to hell" message and I didn't get the joke. "Wait a minute," I thought dully, "I thought we didn't want people to go to hell." And because I didn't think it was funny, did that mean I didn't get Chris anymore? Was I becoming something I never imagined being: utterly humorless?

I didn't know how to deal with any of that. I didn't say anything, turned away from him, packed up my chair and walked to nearby conservation land feeling immense sadness on many levels. I had changed so much, and my brain injury was starting to affect my relationships with the people who mattered most to me.

Chris weighs in on being the son of a survivor

After he worked with me for many months to produce the video "You Look Great! – Inside a Traumatic Brain Injury," I asked Chris what advice he'd offer the children of survivors. He wrote:

> We have only vague, theoretical insights into what it's like to have mild TBI. If you think you find yourself getting frustrated at what seems like your [injured] father's "incompetence" or his defeatist attitude, imagine the self-imposed guilt that he is heaping upon himself for having these shortcomings in the first place.
>
> You should assume that on a daily basis, every person with whom he interacts (whether they are aware of the injury or not) makes him feel like he's screwing up in some way or another. It's up to you to pick up the slack, and to be discreet about there being any "slack" in the first place.

Your children will likely worry about you in ways that show they are very much tuned in to the effects of mild TBI. Chris added:

> I worry about the meds he is prescribed. I worry about the restrictions imposed by the injury becoming more habitual, and that instead of feeling positive about an eventual recovery he might just become reflexively prone to "not being able to handle things," and for his

> injury to so significantly (psychologically) alter/weaken coping mechanisms that need to be exercised, he'll stop recognizing how to effectively deal with things emotionally, socially, etc.

All three of our sons are keenly aware that the injury has altered their relationship with me. Chris reminded me that one of the things that he and Andrew used to do before my injury was to mess with me by hitting my "pressure points" and then informing me that they were being "funny" at my expense:

> This used to be more or less acceptable, but since Dad lacks a lot of his old coping mechanisms (which require a certain capacity for multi-tasking), now this basically just frustrates him, and then further frustrates him that he feels like we're under the impression that he "can't take a joke." Which he can: He's usually up for a good ribbing and is the same ironic, irreverent, and self-effacing dude he's always been. It's just that we can't quite "push the envelope" as far or as often as we once did, which is maybe a good thing.

Our children are aware of each other's efforts to help me, and do make efforts to make everyday life easier for me and Lynne.

Worries

Children can be very perceptive about the changes in household and family dynamics that TBI produces. Like me, my sons fret about the effects of my injury on Lynne. "My mom is responsible for much more now and sometimes seems depressed or stressed," Chris says.

They also worry about Will, their kid brother. Chris characterizes Will as "a rock star and a sports babe who seems like a happy teenager for the most part," but Chris says it would be helpful for Will "to have a Dad who had the energy to be more assertive." They also know that I regret being injured when Will was only 12 years old. Chris says:

> It's sometimes difficult for me to remember how my Dad "used to be" (I am not suggesting that his personality has changed at all), but I know it's even harder for Will.
>
> My Dad told me he knows he would have played a lot more guitar with Will, who started playing (I think) right around the time of the accident. They still play together, but my Dad doesn't even plug in by himself very often anymore. It requires too much energy, and the fact that it takes him exponentially longer to execute day-to-day tasks leaves him little time to do something that would drain him cognitively in any way.

This leads to an important point. Children do have anxieties about a parent with TBI. Will suffers from clinical anxiety, has trouble sleeping, and endures terrible migraines, and I'd be lying if I said I haven't wondered if Will's challenges are somehow associated with my TBI or Andrew's painful back injury.

When asked if any good has come out of all of this – my and Andrew's partial recovery from injuries – Chris warmed my heart and brought me great peace when he responded:

> SO MUCH good has come from this injury. Obviously, it's brought us all closer, and at least in comparison to many of my friends' families, we are the tightest-knit of them all. My Dad is my best friend.

Developing positive attitudes and behaviors

Expanding on Chris's optimism, children *can* develop some truly positive attitudes and behaviors as a result of having a parent with TBI. In our case, these include the following:

- They learn patience and how to cope with frustration and change;

- They become more tolerant, empathetic, considerate, and responsible;

- They discover problem-solving skills they didn't know they possessed;

- They serve willingly as role models for younger siblings;

- They discover that some good can come out of bad circumstances;

- They exhibit less of the narcissistic behavior "typical" of teens;

- They mature socially as they "pick up the slack" for the injured parent;

- They are inspired to build on the positive attitudes of the injured parent;

- They see that a disabled person can have a fulfilling life and purpose;

- They recognize the importance and strength of the family.

After reading this list, Andrew noted, "These are changes and qualities that children *should* adopt. We all fall short when dealing with a parent's TBI."

Getting "TBI smart"

Given the amount of time we spend with our families, their role as support group and recovery team is critical. And don't allow your role as loving parent to be a casualty of the injury. In fact, spouse, survivor, and children can all take action to overcome and manage the enormous strain TBI puts on a family.

Andrew and Will's strategies below and on the next few pages reinforce my conviction that a parent's TBI can lead to children's growth; they illustrate that kids can definitely get "TBI smart."

ANDREW'S STRATEGIES FOR CHILDREN OF TBI SURVIVORS

Strategy	Example or Explanation
Behaviors to avoid:	
Don't ask, "How are you feeling today?"	This is an open-ended question that's hard for my Dad to answer, but more importantly, if I ask it all the time it's like constantly reminding him of his injury. It's more helpful for me to be supportive in other ways that make him feel like a Dad instead of an injured person. I want him to know that he is still very much someone I can turn to, and regularly asking him, "How are you feeling today?" might make him feel like a delicate "case."
Don't be confrontational	You'll continue to disagree with your injured parent about one thing or another, but being aggressively confrontational won't get you anywhere. Survivors find it hard to argue, even about impersonal subjects. In the heat of the moment find a way to back off and let disagreements slide. Figure out a way to discuss it later in a balanced, considerate way.

Strategy	Example or Explanation
Adapt to the new realities of both parents:	
Allow your injured mother or father to parent you	One of the best ways you can show support is to seek guidance from your injured parent. My Dad has always thought that parenting is his most important job, so if I give him plenty of opportunities to parent me, it helps him feel better about himself. Your injured parent will know that you are turning to him less often, and if your parent is anything like my Dad, this will be painful. I try to find a balance between involving Dad in my issues and trying to shield him from them, and sometimes that's a tightrope walk.
Recognize that your non-injured parent is going to carry more burdens.	My mom does even more since Dad sustained his injury, so I try to help her out as much as I can.
Show consideration:	
Be quieter	Noise aggravates my Dad's cognitive problems, so I've learned to lower the volume of my music and to keep my friends quieter. I even try to unload the dishwasher as quietly as I can.
When you invite your friends over, make sure they accommodate the needs of your injured parent	I figure that it's really important to try to live as normally as I did before Dad's injury, and that means I continue to have my friends to the house like I did before. For one thing, I know that my mom likes to have my friends around. For another, I like to have kids to my house. I just try to have them be extra considerate by confining the wrestling and the really loud stuff to the outdoors. There are times when I know my Dad is having a particularly hard day and I don't want him to have to retreat to get away from us. My friends understand.

Strategy	Example or Explanation
Put your support into action:	
Stay on top of your injured parent's treatment	When my Dad talks about a visit to Spaulding Rehab I always listen carefully so I know what's going on, although a lot of times the best thing for Dad is to avoid conversation. If he is cognitively tired after a treatment or appointment, I try to find out from Mom about what's current with him – it's one less thing he needs to say. TBI really affects parent-child communication and it's easy for a gap to form. I make a conscious effort to stay close to Dad and to keep myself updated about his recovery efforts. It's a way to show my support.
Take on more responsibility	You need to know that you will have to start handling more things yourself. I took a year off from college in part because I needed a break, but I also wanted to be around the house more to help with my younger brother and to do whatever needed doing. I did make a difference – even if on certain days I was only cleaning the kitchen or driving Will somewhere.
Learn your injured parent's "triggers"	Noise is difficult for my Dad, so I am always trying to minimize it. Also, since he can feel overwhelmed by detail, I try to present stuff (such as a paper I want him to read or a story I want to tell him) in an organized and simple way, without a lot of loose ends.
Communicate with your siblings:	
Share your insights with family members	TBI – especially mild TBI – is a very confusing injury. The parent looks the same so it's hard to "translate" why he would be acting so differently. If you have younger siblings who just don't get why, try to explain as best you can what is going on and reinforce his understanding when possible. Also, if you discover something helpful – like a certain way of communicating that seems to work – share it with your brothers, sisters, and non-injured parent. When it's appropriate, confirm it with your injured parent.

Strategy	Example or Explanation
Respect your injured parent's new reality:	
You can hope that something good will come out of your parent's brain injury, but never think of it as a blessing in disguise and never say that it is	You hear stories about people losing a leg or an eye or having some other injury and then they bounce back with best-selling memoirs where they say they'd never trade the injury for their former life. This book came out of my Dad's injury and it is something positive. And, he would say that the injury has made him stronger in some ways. But he would trade the injury for his old life in a heartbeat. Day to day life is so much harder for a person with mild TBI – Dad feels sick most of the time – and it's very hard for me to hear people say that it's a "blessing." It's a very easy thing for someone who doesn't have the injury to say that, but it's ignorant.

WILL'S STRATEGIES FOR CHILDREN OF TBI SURVIVORS

Strategy	Example or Explanation
Handle chaotic social interactions when you can	I traveled to Kansas with my Dad to spend time with my grandmother and other relatives and I knew Dad would enjoy it, but that it would be hard for him. I told him I could handle things on my own when he needed to be by himself and lie down. I made an effort to interact with everybody when he couldn't. Generally I try to be as energetic as I can, even if I'm in a bad mood, and try to do more of the talking so Dad doesn't have to.
Plan ahead and schedule events around your parents	Dad has to allot his time carefully because of his injury so I don't want to throw any curve balls into his day. I let him know ahead of time when I have plans. I can't say, "Oh, I'm having friends over in an hour." Instead I'll say I'm having friends over next Tuesday. It's hard to plan ahead when you're not used to it, but in the long run it's a good skill to stay ahead of the game. I try to plan my own schedule around my parents' plans.
Minimize your frustration with a brain-injured parent by thinking about the injury in a helpful way	Getting frustrated at somebody with a brain injury is like getting frustrated at somebody who is missing a leg and can't walk as fast as you can.
Problem-solve	I was 12 when Dad got injured and in the fifth grade I would ask him to help me solve a computer problem. I'm 17 now and try to figure stuff out by myself. Even though I know he's happy to help me, I know he'd feel crappy later on. So to open up Dad's day I try my best to be as independent as I can to make things as easy as possible for him and for my mother. You find out by yourself what these things are. Problem-solving on your own is not a bad thing.

Strategy	Example or Explanation
Know that you will mature quicker	I have learned to be as independent as I can because TBI changes the parent who is injured and the dynamic of a family. It's not the end of the world, but things will be harder for everybody than they were before. So taking responsibility for things – even something that's not a big deal, like cleaning up the kitchen – makes things easier for everybody.
Learn how to interpret your parent's behavior correctly	Your injured parent can't do what he did before. You have to realize that he's not being lazy if he is taking naps or resting. The batteries of people with TBI are weaker than ours and they have to "recharge."
Help to reduce your injured parent's stress	Stress drains anybody's battery, but it can empty the battery of a person with TBI. If you can limit the stress in an injured parent's life, that's the best thing you can do. Here are some of the things I do: • If I want to have a conversation with Dad, I try to have it in a quiet place where there is no background noise or multiple conversations. • I tell my friends to keep their noise to a minimum. • My friends aren't as conscious of Dad's challenges as I am, but when I tell them to stop something–say a friend is on a bouncy ball–they cut it out.
Recognize that the world doesn't revolve around you	TBI will make things "not normal." I think it's probably normal for a teenager to be self-absorbed, but TBI forces you to think about other family members in a way that may be less self-centered than in "normal" families. This is probably a good thing.

Strategy	Example or Explanation
Remember that you're a role model for any younger sisters and/or brothers	Your little sister or little brother has definitely lost something. Take it upon yourself to pick up the slack and change that.
It's okay to be angry about your parent's injury	It's okay if you're angry that your parent got injured – I think there's a lot of anger about TBI, especially for a kid – but if your injured parent is angry and bitter, nothing good is going to come out of it. My Dad has taken it upon himself to help others with TBI, so a lot of good has come out of it. That has helped me.
Be upbeat	Be as positive as you can. It will make your injured parent feel better.
Help your injured parent when you travel together	Do what you can to support your parent when you travel because no matter what, he will feel exhausted when you get to your destination and will need a day or so to recuperate. Traveling is hard and you just have to help your parent get through it.

24 – The Possible Role of Prayer in Recovery

KEEPING AN OPEN MIND ABOUT PRAYER

I would be seriously remiss if I left out one of the most important parts of my recovery: praying during my darkest times. Some have suggested that I should leave out any mention of God in this book because it might offend or even repel a part of my audience. I considered this of course, but in the end I had to conclude that praying has served as a key strategy in dealing with this injury and, since this book seeks to compile strategies, it is necessary to bring up.

I would caution people who might be turned off by this particular thread to think of the strategy open-mindedly, the way a skeptic of holistic medicine should still consider the possible benefits of acupuncture and dietary supplements. As I say at various points throughout this book, desperate times call for desperate measures.

Prayer as strategy

With TBI, the sights and sounds of this world are going to drive you to a dark place, both physically and psychically. Frankly, you are probably going to feel the need to be alone a lot during your recovery. While this self-imposed exile from friends and family will intensify your loneliness, it can also be an incredibly valuable time of spiritual reflection, meditation, and reaching out into the mysteries of the Divine.

In the interest of your recovery, I encourage you to keep an open mind and consider several things:

- Attack this injury and your recovery from as many vantage points possible. This will mean trying things that you might initially feel skeptical about, such as support groups, acupuncture, craniosacral therapy, or neuropsychology.

- Accept graciously if people offer to pray for you. Even though he had no conviction it would do him any good, even Christopher Hitchens, the world's most famous atheist, never told people not to pray for him during his battle with esophageal cancer.

- Engaging in prayer for your family, friends, and your fellow survivors at the very least temporarily takes your attention off of yourself. It will also remind you of the needs of others during a time when you will tend to be self-absorbed. This in itself can stave off depression.

PRAYERS OF DESPERATION

The Bible insists that God hears the prayers of the desperate

"I called upon thy name, O Lord, out of the low dungeon." Lamentations 3:55

I said that desperate times call for desperate measures. Obviously, your life with TBI qualifies as desperate times. If you're like me, you have experienced times when you've felt so bad that as you lay there you held out your arm and fantasized that someone would inject something that would make you feel good. You do not think this would be too much to ask or expect.

So, given our desperation, one way to begin this act of prayer is to ask not once, but repeatedly: "Now what, God?" In so doing, we take this incredible burden that we bear and lift it up to Him. In effect we are challenging Him to show us what our lives have been saved for.

Of course it is not possible to shame God, any more than the Prophets did in Scripture when they cried out things like, "How long, O Lord? How long will you keep your face turned from your people?" But when I lie down and am not sleeping and can't even move – all I can do is breathe – I breathe deliberately. Sometimes I breathe a series of prayers. With each exhale I think, "Oh . . . God . . . have . . . mercy . . . on . . . me . . ." or if I am feeling inclusive, I end with "us," including my fellow survivors.

And if I don't want my brain to recite even that many words, I inhale and then pray just one word on the exhale, as though I have my arm twisted behind my back with my tormentor waiting for that word. I pray simply, "Mercy . . ." [inhale] "Mercy . . ." ad infinitum, so in effect – at least I hope this is the effect – the onus is on God to show me His mercy and relieve me of this misery. To up the ante, after a series of "Mercy," which I pray simply to stop the misery, I begin a series of "Grace," by which I mean, "And bless me, too!" Your move.

Call it the power of suggestion if you like, but I am calling it the power of prayer. From my wounded, pinned-down, shot-at position, I am calling for reinforcements. I am calling for Reinforcement. I am calling in the big guns. I am calling in the Big Gun. I am calling in air strikes against the enemy. And HQ does not take such battlefield requests lightly.

One day I read this in the book of Lamentations:

> Thou hast heard my voice: hide not thine ear at my breathing, at my cry. Thou drewest near in the day that I called upon thee: thou saidst, Fear not. O Lord, thou hast pleaded the causes of my soul; thou hast redeemed my life. (3:56-58)

So I have it on good Authority that this breathing-and-praying method is paying off.

The Psalms

Throughout my recovery I have felt great affinity with the authors of the 150 Psalms. Theirs was not a cushioned faith; they literally faced death and called on the only One they knew could hear them and answer them. Many times David, one of the authors, wrote in great desperation, sitting in a cave surrounded by his warrior enemies. What he wrote as physical reality, survivors can interpret as metaphor, and in our desperation we need hold nothing back from our prayers.

Consider Psalm 57:

> Be merciful to me, O God, be merciful to me; for my soul trusts in Thee.
>
> Yea, in the shadow of Thy wings will I make my refuge, until these calamities be overpast.
>
> I will cry unto God Most High; unto God who performeth all things for me.
>
> He shall send from heaven and save me from the reproach of him who would swallow me up. God shall send forth His mercy and His truth.

"Cover my defenseless head . . ."

One Sunday morning our church congregation sang a hymn that was new to me. When we got to the second verse, I sang robustly:

> Other refuge have I none; Hangs my helpless soul on Thee.
> Leave, ah, leave me not alone, still support and comfort me!

> All my trust on Thee is stayed, all my help from Thee I bring;
> Cover my defenseless head with the shadow of Thy wing.

No matter what your faith, I encourage you to connect your suffering to the suffering of "your people," whoever they might be; for example:

- If you are a Christian, stare at a crucifix and reflect on – and possibly discover – your special relationship to the suffering and now risen Christ.

- If you are Jewish, stare at and reflect on the Star of David. Consider your Jewish brothers and sisters in Europe in the 1930s and 40s, and the gathering together in 1948 to create the nation of Israel.

- If you are Muslim, consider the violence and suffering between and among your Sunni and Shiite brothers and sisters, not to mention the plight of the Palestinians, and pray for peace. We must all pray for peace.

If you have not been a believing or praying person to this point, as you lie there or sit there in your suffering, imagine as vividly as your pain a loving God there with you. If you want to smile, think of God saying in a mother's voice, "Would it kill you to call home once in awhile?"

❧ ❧

Of the three phases of TBI recovery – Awareness, Adjustment, Acceptance – the last is the hardest to talk about and come to grips with. Author Kathleen Casey Theisen, is more hard-nosed and practical than many when trying to come to grips with what acceptance means: "Acceptance is not submission; it is acknowledgement of the facts of a situation. Then deciding what you're going to do about it." True acceptance of "this hand we've been dealt," as Mike puts it, is elusive, but it begins with recognizing certain milestones of recovery, each of which tests our resolve to accept our new lives.

ACCEPTANCE

"The pages are still blank, but there is a miraculous feeling

of the words being there, written in invisible ink

and clamoring to become visible."

Vladimir Nabokov

25 – Dragging Your Injury to Milestones

DRAGGING YOUR INJURY AROUND WITH YOU

Survivors of all stripes – TBI, cancer, spurned or lost love – know how elusive acceptance can be. We know that no matter where we are, we drag our injury around with us. Even with time away from jobs, living with a brain injury is not, as somebody said to a friend of mine, like having an extended vacation.

. . . even to paradise

This is never clearer to me than when I head to our remote, low-tech cabin in Maine for the sole purpose of not talking. Talking is one of the most taxing things I do. Sometimes I just sit on the dock and stare at the water. I watch when the wind blows the water silently, and from all directions. I watch when the sun lights up the rippling surfaces of the water like at a World Series night game when somebody hits a home run.

The great thing about Maine is I listen only to what my brain needs; I sleep and rest when I have to, and not just when I can "slip away." Sometimes I'll get up in the morning and not do anything more taxing than make breakfast, eat it, and read something, and two hours later my eyes sag and my brain starts to shut down. If I walk by a mirror I look like I'm dying. As quiet and peaceful as Maine is, I have dragged my injury there with me.

TRAVELING LIGHTLY

Given this great weight that we drag with us, we need to otherwise travel as lightly as possible.

Figure 10:

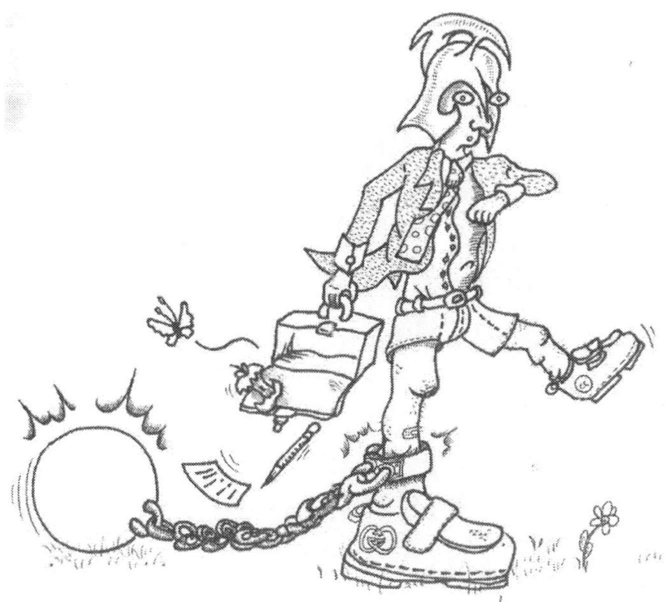

Artwork: Chris Byler

Traveling lightly will mean many things, and making use of many strategies, but at a minimum it will mean:

- Relinquishing some responsibilities, and

- Resolving our anger at what has happened to us.

Relinquishing responsibilities

Although a doctor might tell you this doesn't make sense, many survivors will tell you that as time goes on – say into your third and fourth year – you might find that you're unable to do some things you could do earlier in your recovery. You notice areas of improvement, even in stops and starts, but don't be surprised if you look back in your journal or "progress notes" and say, "I could never do all that now!"

Actually, I think it's more a matter of, "I *would* never do all that now!" You might just be learning to pace yourself better and not over-extend yourself. Many survivors agree that this is especially hard for people who are used to being high-performing before their injuries, whether in their careers – lots of promotions – or even in their choice of hobbies, as in the case of marathoners. But this is a key aspect of trying to recover from a brain injury: having the discipline to relinquish unnecessary responsibilities that drain you.

Figuring out your "critical path"

Project managers use a tool called the critical path method. It helps them figure out what tasks directly contribute to the project, and what tasks slow down or otherwise hurt the project in some way; for example, tasks that are redundant or expensive. Obviously, the more clearly the project manager identifies both kinds of tasks – *and acts on those findings* – the more likely it is that the project will be a success.

Through painful trial and error, a process that has continued into my sixth year of recovery, you too will learn to relinquish taxing responsibilities that are not in your critical path. Survivors need to identify responsibilities that are absolutely core to who they are and what they deem most important in their lives. It might be family for one survivor, it might be family *and* friends for another, and it might be only self-preservation for another.

I tried serving on the board of a small local charity, but as my first two-hour meeting wore on I knew I was going to pay a price the next day. Although I felt I was making a reasonable contribution to the meeting, I found it hard to keep track of what people were saying, and if I thought of something to say I had to struggle to remember it on my frail "cognitive clipboard" while waiting for a chance to actually say it. This meant I couldn't pay close attention to what was being said.

Sure enough, the next day I felt terrible. I'd overheated my brain. I had to decide that this charity was not on my critical path to my recovery. I reluctantly wrote them this e-mail, and although I felt like I was letting them down, I knew it was the right thing to do:

> Hello Board members,
> I've got to step down already from the Board. Believe me, I regret having to do this. I thought I could be helpful or useful but the past month has been so hard, and it's simply because I persist in "doing too much," a lot of which you guys probably do for leisure: dinner with friends, and so on. I think I'm setting myself up to 1) let the Board down, and 2) set back my so-called recovery.

I include this anecdote because most days survivors face hard choices. On the one hand, you want to be a valuable and valued human being, and often that requires cognitive effort. On the other hand, you want to recover as fully as possible from your brain injury, and that requires resting your brain, shielding it from excessive stimulation. Consider which cognitive efforts are worth the harsh aftermath, and make your choices with care.

And if you decide you can't or shouldn't do something on a particular day, knowing which tasks are on and off your critical path to recovery absolves you from feeling guilty about it. This is no small thing. Guilt feelings can really wear you down, and can lead to depression, which is *not* on your critical path!

I have since gone on to serve on the board of the BIA-MA, and am learning ways of getting through those meetings. One way is to think back to the lawnmower metaphor I've used: using my brain is like mowing a patch of long, wet grass. In meetings, I keep the mower running when I need to and then during stretches when my concentration is not required – say, during financial reports – I shut the mower off. I coast. Coasting, in fact, is an under-reported strategy for survivors, whether in meetings or in everyday conversation. In a sense, the "critical path" is the only one that needs mowing.

One time I told Rick Sanders about playing my guitar again, which I took fairly seriously before the injury. I was finding it therapeutic but also exhausting. He asked me, "Do you find playing the guitar draining?" As with so many questions Rick has asked me, this was an interesting one. I hesitated before I answered because it must be like if you're recovering from a heart attack and the doctor asks if you find having sex physically strenuous. "Please," you're thinking, "don't take that away from me." I admitted that it was draining, but that it was worth it. Now I consider playing my guitar to be on my critical path. It just plays a different part in my recovery.

Resolving anger

"Resentment kills a fool, and envy slays the simple." Job 5:2

Looking to come up with a list of feelings, at one support-group meeting someone asked us, "How do you *feel* as you try to recover from your brain injury?" Various words were offered, such as "hopeful" or "frustrated," but I noticed that nobody mentioned anger or resentment.

I commended the group for not bringing that up even though for most of us it would have been easy to. Although we inevitably drag our injury around with us wherever we go, we should not drag all the other baggage that comes with our "incident." Many people's injuries, like mine, came as a result of someone else's actions, whether intentional or not. Those of us hit in cars by maniacs or drunks – or drunk maniacs – could end up seething perpetually in anger.

I told them I'd seen a terrific chart in the *New York Times* that showed the distinct lack of progress made by patients who used up energy by letting anger and resentment fester. But the best way to describe the toxic effects came from Carrie Fisher and her one-woman show, Wishful Drinking. She said, "Resentment is like drinking a poison and hoping that the other person dies."

Arguing with the ref

We've all seen in professional sports when a referee or an umpire makes a bad call on one of the players – or at least the player believes it is a bad call – and the player gets so worked up about it that he forgets to get back in the game. The game is going on around him, and the other team might even be scoring points or runs while he argues. While we must stand up for ourselves and even get legal help if someone is responsible for our injury, there will come a time when we have to get our head back into the game so life does not pass us by.

The power of forgiveness

But anger might come, and if it does, consider the power of forgiveness. You might even look at it as not giving the reckless jackass who hit you the satisfaction of a moment's more thought. As my mother wrote in an essay on love:

> Do you know someone unlovable? Or who has hurt you? I discovered a long time ago that if I cannot forgive someone, I cannot be lovable. If I am neither loving nor lovable, I would turn into a bitter person. There would be dark spots on my personality much like an overripe banana.

A friend of mine was asked to prepare and conduct an 18-week Sunday School class on forgiveness. At first he thought, "What are we going to talk about after about the third class?" He told me later that the subject of forgiveness was so compelling and rich that, even after 18 weeks, they actually ran out of time.

The impossibility of real justice

A survivor I know sat in his lawyer's conference room while a mediator worked his way through the details of the case with both sets of lawyers. Things grew heated when the insurance company's lawyer repeatedly refused to acknowledge the liability of his client and the severity of my friend's injury – which included his inability to now have children. The settlement, which on the surface might seem like a large amount, only included the prorated cost of the survivor's medications for the rest of his life.

The mediator assigned both parties to a separate room, and came in to speak with my friend and his wife. Here is the essence of what the mediator said:

> Let's say this accident never happened. We fast-forward to five years from now, and you and your wife have two children. A man knocks on your door and says he will give you a million dollars, but he will take both your children, beat you up, leaving you with a brain injury, and wreak havoc on every aspect of your life. What would you say to him?
>
> My friend and his wife said no, of course they would not accept the man's offer. The mediator paused to let all of this sink in, and then said, "I just want you to realize that, given all that has happened to you, no matter how this case goes, you will not receive justice. Nothing can give you back what you have lost.

Forgiving someone who caused your injury could well be a crucial part of your recovery, as could a realization that true justice is impossible, even with someone responsible for your misery sitting behind bars. Stewing in bitterness, anger, and resentment is a terrible environment in which to heal your brain, and it won't alleviate your depression or improve the quality of your life. These draining, toxic emotions are not on your critical path to recovery.

The major victory far exceeded the small defeat

The ceremonies of which I was master

Before the injury, one of my strong suits was serving as Master of Ceremonies for fundraising banquets of 250 guests for a few charities that mean a lot to me. I was asked to host one over a year after the accident, and I presented the challenge to Rick Sanders. I said I really wanted to try it again, partly because I missed being good at something.

He had me start the writing process months in advance, something that before the injury had taken me several days. I wrote slowly and in short sessions, feeling the strain I was placing on my brain. But when I wrote the funny parts, the process sometimes gave me actual pleasure. I proudly showed Rick my drafts, and as the date drew near I rehearsed over and over again, not leaving even a word to chance.

I must say I MC'd the banquet flawlessly. I had not stammered at all because I had my entire script in front of me. I felt in control of my performance, and I cannot describe the pleasure I felt looking out at all those smiling faces. Then something interesting happened. I stepped down from podium and talked with my friend Joe, who complimented me.

Joe is a wonderful pianist and I eagerly told him about my new piano lessons. But as I tried to speak, I started stammering badly and I couldn't continue the conversation. There was something about the complicated subject of music, a topic dear to both of us, and trying to find the words for the differences between playing the guitar instinctively by ear and learning to read music to play the piano. Trying to find the right words, especially over background noise, was all much too much for me. Just at the moment I should have been savoring a success, I felt I'd been punched in the stomach.

Paying the TBI piper

It occurred to me on the way home that anyone attending the banquet might well have thought, "You say he has a brain injury? Boy, I couldn't tell." But for the next five days I had a horrible cognitive hangover. The first day, I crashed on the couch, and in fact I must have looked comical with my C-pap on, earplugs in, noise-canceling headphones on, and the hood from my red sweatshirt pulled over my face.

But performing as MC had made me feel competent and confident, something I hadn't felt in over a year.

The annual banquet is in my critical path

The evening of the fundraiser was a turning point for me. Despite the effort involved and the cost of my recovery, I felt real pride in the quality of my writing and delivery. I also felt a surge of adrenaline at holding the attention of that many people, and having them smile up at me, and sometimes even laugh. This is something I wanted to do once a year, assuming I would be asked to do it again. (I was, and I did.)

THREE KINDS OF MILESTONES

I almost called this chapter, "Passing Your Milestones like Kidney Stones," but I realized that survivors pass three kinds of milestones, and they don't have to be painful. You should record all of them in your journal:

1. Anniversary milestones

An anniversary milestone might begin with "I sustained my injury one month ago today," but then before we know it, if the injury does not go away, we mark our first and second anniversaries and beyond. The reality and possible permanence of the injury begins to set in, and we commit to major adjustments in our new lives.

2. Significant-event milestones

These milestones mark both bad and good events in your recovery. The bad milestones are examples of the reality of your injury. These include specific sequelae that you experience, as well as the aftermath of your cognitive exertions. For example:

- "Today I realized I cannot spend more than 20 minutes in a grocery store," or even more specifically, "Today I realized I should not spend ten minutes deciding which peanut butter to buy."

The good milestones mark specific improvements in your cognition and quality of life, the encouraging turning points and personal breakthroughs of your recovery.

3. Moving-toward-acceptance milestones

These milestones mark the junctures in our recovery that tell us that we might be moving towards acceptance. These specific incidents, even if they are inadvertent – if something slips out of your mouth that speaks of something you didn't know was in your heart – show that you might be moving from denial or bitterness about your injury to a much healthier place. You might be approaching that elusive stage of recovery called acceptance – acceptance of your injury and of your new life that stretches out in front of you.

A milestone on the way to acceptance

Sometimes the first thing out of your mouth is the truest thing.

In the middle of a weekday afternoon I drove to the post office, in no particular hurry because I had plenty of time before it closed. As usual I was feeling terrible from the injury. Up ahead I saw a school bus stopped and I realized school had just let out. I stopped and waited for a couple of children to step out of the bus and cross the street.

As the bus started up again and I drove past it, I saw a line of cars slowly starting to move too. Most of the drivers looked stressed and impatient and frustrated – they looked as though they were cursing their rotten luck that they'd gotten stuck behind a school bus. Some had rolled their windows down so they could crane their necks out and see what the holdup was. Some were even looking at their watches.

In an instant I remembered the stresses of absolutely having to be somewhere and running late and then having to stop behind a school bus on top of it all. As I drove past them I spontaneously said, "There but for the grace of God go I."

That really hit me. I thought, "Is this acceptance?"

Many survivors have moments like these, and while they usually don't mean you've finally come to grips with everything that's unraveled in your life, it is a brief moment of peace. And sometimes these moments come with something that feels like hope, a sense of assurance in our hearts that we are in good hands after all.

In this chapter I've encouraged you to keep track during your recovery of important turning points and personal breakthroughs, and relieve yourself of unnecessary burdens. Before moving on to the final chapter, we should at least touch on – skate on the surface of – the issue of suffering. It will serve as a transition to the eyes-wide-open conclusion: Living This New Life.

26 – The Divine Mean vs. Divine Meanness

DIVINE MEAN

The "Divine Mean," also called the Divine Proportion, Golden Mean, or Phi, refers to balance and proportion; simple patterns found in nature and used in science, architecture, and art. If the survivor is open to positive and constructive interpretations in life, we can try to see an injury like TBI as bringing balance to our lives, lives that might have been too obsessed with career or otherwise funding one's 401(k).

But most of the time we're in no mood to hear about blessings in disguise or how this might have been the best thing to have ever happened to us. Please. If there are lessons to be learned from bearing this injury, they are never tutorials, they are always self-study. Even though people mean well, they really do, they should leave us to work this thing out. We can always turn to the survivor seated next to us in this class and confer.

DIVINE MEANNESS

"Divine Mean," if you are free-associating, can also make you think "God is mean" or "Divine meanness," also known as theodicy, the age-old question of how a good God can allow suffering and evil.

People have asked me, "Aren't you mad at God?" and I've got to say that when you and your son walk away from a totaled car you're grateful. Over the years as we've raised our children, bad things have happened to people in the world and to our own family and friends. So in light of the tragedies of this world –

whether it's collateral damage in war, earthquakes in Japan, floods in New Orleans, genocide in Darfur, or malignant cancer in my father and brother – the question is not so much, "Why me?" but "Why not me?" Before the injury I don't recall ever thinking, "I have a great life! Why me?"

We want to be protected, not just eternally, but here and now. But anyone who has read Ecclesiastes knows that life isn't fair or just, and that:

> The race is not to the swift, and the battle is not to the warriors, and neither is bread to the wise, nor wealth to the discerning, nor favor to men of ability. *(Ecclesiastes 9:11)*

Sure, this is not the life I envisioned for myself. It's too embarrassing and humbling, for one thing. But is this the life you envisioned for yourself? Are we really in charge of our lives? Ask yourself that hard question, and let me give you my two cents.

WHAT TO MAKE OF SUFFERING

Who does God choose to reveal Himself to? According to the Psalms, "The Lord is close to the brokenhearted and saves those who are crushed in spirit" (34:18); and "The Lord preserves the simple; I was brought low, and He saved me." (116:6) That God reveals Himself to the broken and the simple is good news for many of us recovering from a brain injury.

I spoke at a grad school about the injury, and a student asked, "Were you spiritual before the accident?" I said I didn't think that I'm especially spiritual now – I think about food a lot, for example – but if she meant God-fearing then yes I was before and I am now. After some not-very-withering cross-examination I warmed to the topic and told her that nothing should surprise us and nothing should shake our faith in God. Are we under some illusion as to who God is and what to expect from this life? Did we think that we could sidestep tragedy in this life?

"Life is suffering" is incomplete

As I spoke to many survivors and as I went through my journals in the writing of this book, I came across many instances of hope-deflating, life-sapping suffering. Here's an example, which really got me thinking:

> Tried to reconcile/accept the fact of living with suffering . . . and doing what I have to do or need to do or want to do. Not to pursue suffering but not shrink from it if "duty calls."

I wrote that in my journal because I felt strongly that the Buddhist maxim "life is suffering" is incomplete. I think it is intended to prepare us for the inevitability of suffering so that we're not surprised or caught up short when it happens to us, but if that statement is the sum total of our philosophy of suffering, it can too easily lead to cynicism, and even nihilism and despair. I felt that brain injury survivors have to resist all of that and treat them like we would any other toxins that would invade our systems. A brain injury makes you hyper-aware of what truly motivates you to press on and what discourages you to the point of depression.

To look at life honestly, it is truer to say that life *includes* suffering – that goes without saying – and that life is also so much more. Life is also overcoming adversity, being graceful under pressure, easing someone else's suffering, and, God help us, not surrendering to our circumstances.

In these grave times of recovery our lives are placed in stark contrast with the lives of most other people. As Gregg put it in an early chapter when I asked bitterly why I couldn't even enjoy casually reading a novel like most people: "John, we're not like most people."

Then who are we? Are we survivors only, or can we be more than just survivors?

TAKING RICK'S ADVICE

In the previous chapter I mentioned dragging my injury to the benign, healing environment of our Maine cabin. I confessed these feelings of frustration to Rick Sanders, and even feelings of guilt for not savoring that paradise. He said something that has stayed with me ever since:

> You have to figure out and decide how to live the rest of your life.

In the final chapter, we'll try to take Rick's advice, and figure out and decide how to live the rest of our lives. We'll look at some ways of interpreting what has happened to us, and the role acceptance plays in how to live this new life.

27 – Living This New Life

"Why is life given to a man whose way is hidden, whom God has hedged in?"
Job 3:23

YOU SURVIVED. NOW WHAT?

You and I are survivors. However we choose to interpret our accident or our incident, and however far along we might have come in our recovery, the fact is that we survived what could easily have been the final, fatal chapter in our story. We are alive. Blood courses through our veins. Our temples and our pulses throb. We think thoughts and have desires. We even dare to have dreams and aspirations. Because dead people cannot say the same thing, the obvious fact of our continued existence is an excellent place to discuss living this new life of ours.

Living these fast lives in the breakdown lane

What is next for us? For many survivors, I would even say for most survivors, each day has its share of rough times, physically, emotionally and, needless to say, cognitively. Each day has dark moments that often stretch into hours. Should we face the rest of our day and each tomorrow in fear and dread and resignation? Or should we find ways to get through our rough times and live to fight the good fight another day?

Each day we must learn how to overcome what has happened to us. We begin by accepting the reality of our new lives and believing in the possibilities of a rich future. This acceptance is usually incremental, and we've looked at some milestones along the way. We dream and hope in the long term but we actually live these new lives in the short term, day after excruciating day. So if we do not quite accept the suffering as it's happening, we have to work as though our lives depend on applying strategies to each difficulty. And of course they do.

This final chapter suggests some ways to live this new life, and I hope it encourages you to:

- Never give up.

- Never shrink to the dimensions of your disability.

- Find ways to break the bondage of your injury.

- Always fight loneliness and depression.

- Take time to find pleasure in your new life.

- Never apologize to anyone for having an injury.

- Find ways to be generous in your poverty, grateful in your infirmity.

To recap: Never give up.

OUR NEW IDENTITY

We are bigger than our injury, and we are more than just survivors

One way we can begin living this new life is to change the way we look at ourselves. We cannot let this injury define who we are, or let it become our identity. For example, my website tbistrategies.com and e-mail address mildTBI@gmail.com are for TBI-related issues only. They do not define me because TBI is not all of who I am.

"Thrive-vivor"

The word survivor connotes different things for different people, and some people with a brain injury do not like to use it. They see themselves as something more than just survivors. My friend Michelle insists she is a "thrive-vivor," meaning that she fully intends to thrive and not simply survive in her new life. Being a strong and sometimes stubborn person, she tends to to prove to herself that she can and will thrive, even if it means overextending herself. For her, this can lead to such painful and debilitating migraines that to find relief she drives over an hour into Boston for a shot of Toradol.

While she is receiving the shot – never a fun moment, she assures me – she is probably calculating all over again, "Now, was that worth it?" She and I can argue good-naturedly about how to answer that question, but what's great is that she does not limit herself by applying the word "survivor" to herself. She is a thrive-vivor.

Whatever we choose to call ourselves, the fact remains that we all survived a possibly fatal incident and many of us have been left in a very similar place in our recovery. Our incident might have been a car accident, an IED explosion, a slip in the bathtub, a blow to the head by a fist or a foot or a fall to hard ground, a stroke or aneurism, or infection, or brain surgery. Often it seems as though our brains have healed up only to a particular point. And this is why support groups can work so effectively. Our reasons for attending might be different, but there we are, sharing strategies and experiences with each other, trying to move from surviving to thrive-viving.

Someone in my brain injury support group referred to me in an e-mail as, "John Byler, the survivor." That took me aback at first, but of course she was right. Seeing "John Byler, the survivor" in virtual print made me feel as though it reduced me to that word, that identity. Just as the statement "life is suffering" is incomplete, so too is the word "survivor." Even though I have used the term throughout this book, we are all, of course, so much more than that. We might also be spouses and partners and parents, friends and colleagues, family and neighbors, and this book has tried to address all the major roles we play in life as we drag our injuries along with us.

Are we castaways or warriors?

The other issue I have with the term "survivor" is that it makes me think of a castaway, someone who a storm has thrown onto an empty and hostile island. Again, we can be so much more than a castaway. We all grapple with this new identity of ours, and we must all make sense of our new surroundings. We must try to find ways – strategies – to re-fashion our environment so that it is friendlier to healing. Think of it as bending the world to our specifications, rather than letting the world bend and break us.

We can see ourselves as castaways only and play the part of victim for the rest of our hard lives. But if it's true that we have escaped death and now suffer the pain of the wreckage – the deprivations and humiliations of living on this island – surely a healthier way of looking at the life of a castaway is that we have fought to establish a beachhead. Beachheads are strategic positions gained through military action; think storming the beaches at Normandy. Those guys didn't stay on the beach. It was death to stay on the beach. Most of them moved inland quickly, and only doubled back to rescue somebody when they felt strong enough to bear the burden of a brother in arms.

So ask yourself these hard questions:

- Am I a survivor and castaway on a beach, or a survivor and warrior who has just established a beachhead?

- Am I a victim or a hero?

- Am I a passive observer of all that has happened to me and is happening all around me, or am I actively shaping these events for my healing and recovery?

You can see how the way we answer these questions affects the way we live our lives, day after difficult day. Maybe you've felt like a victim for too long – the object of one misfortune after another – and you are fed up with your ordeal. Now it is time to see yourself as acting – and having acted throughout your recovery – heroically.

So castaways can define themselves as such, or they can work at making the island habitable. And if they are truly adaptive to their environment, as Darwin said of those who endure, they can one day even thrive.

Learning to thrive on this island

If we choose to take a positive view of ourselves as heroic, we will begin to see that this island beyond the beachhead, while a hostile environment for us, is not barren after all. There is richness here, and fruitfulness, and some of the most profound truths on earth are here. And this island is not as lonely a place as we first thought. If you look for them, you will find other castaways dotting the beaches who at first might not have the strength or the will or the sense of hope to begin exploring.

We can show them how to explore. We can start by giving them a brief tour of some of the hidden treasures, and we can continue exploring the rest of the island together. In my own recovery, after moving inland from my beachhead I established some of the dearest and deepest friendships of my life.

When I am feeling strong, sometimes I go back to the beach – an actual or virtual support group – and carry someone farther inland. If you listen, you can hear them calling out for a medic. That's you. If you go after them, you'll find that they will climb on your shoulders a lot faster than they will for a non-injured caregiver or even a loved one; even someone with a medical degree. You have heard that blood is thicker than water. Sometimes I think that a brain injury is thicker even than blood.

Sacred Journey

When your healing is farther along, and you have been using strategies for living this new life, you will grow stronger. You will have moments of joy again. You will learn to live a life of perpetual restoration, and perhaps even learn to live a playful life. In Frederick Beuchner's memoir, *Sacred Journey*, he writes that his grandmother used to quote her father, Hermann Scharmann: "Never put on your bathing suit without going in the water."

This injury is our bathing suit, and we have been forced to wear it. We must go in the water! From time to time, as often as you can because life is short, allow yourself the luxury of floating on your back and riding the waves. This might mean taking a long walk in a field on a nice day, or putting on headphones and listening to music in a park. If conversation is not too difficult for you, meet a friend in the middle of the day in a beautiful setting for the sole purpose of being together and sharing friendship.

Show the survivors still on the beach what could be in their future if they do not give up. Show them that continued healing is possible, and that using strategies has helped you and will help them. Give them the thing they lack most and need most: hope. Be a leader in the TBI community, and lead by example.

To further reinforce the importance of this new work you are doing – healing, and helping others to heal – consider this as well: Don't give a second thought about the work you used to do or the work your colleagues and friends are doing. Let them build their own sand castles. Time's weather and waves will wash away their temporary constructions.

This isn't meant to be as harsh as that might sound. It is simply a mental image to ward off depression and sadness at what you think you might be missing, and to increase your confidence in what you are doing. Besides all of the emotional and physical agonies of this injury, most of us have also born a terrible financial burden. But I urge you to consider and experience the emotional growth and healing when you work on behalf of others. Your new life can become rich, charitable, satisfying, and may well have a bigger impact on people's lives than what you did every day before your injury.

To recap: Your new life will be worth living.

LIVING THIS NEW LIFE "ALL IN"

The poker metaphor

By any standard, survivors have not exactly been dealt what looks like a winning hand. The deck is clearly stacked against us, and we are not even playing with a full deck. (Stay with me on this.)

Committing to your hand

If you're not familiar with the game of poker, poker players do something called doubling down on their bet. Betting on the hand you've been dealt is one thing, but when you are really confident in that hand you can double your bet.

When you've got what you believe is an unbeatable hand – or when you want the other players to believe you have an unbeatable hand so that they fold – you shove all the money in front of you to the center of the table. It is always a wonderfully cinematic moment. When you believe there's no turning back and the whole game comes down to this play, you are "all in."

It is in those very dark times during my recovery that I've chosen to be like the poker player who says, "I'm all in." I lie there, fully committed to the moment, and with each breath. I say: "I'm all in . . . I'm all in . . . Mercy . . . Mercy." I breathe out to God, "I give up . . . I can't do this on my own . . . Uncle . . . No más . . ." Call it surrender or call it committed, I put the burden on God to bring me relief. Faith is nothing more than trusting in the evidence of things you can't see, and many times we can't see relief ahead. Have faith that your prayers are being heard; that the air you are breathing so prayerfully is bringing you back to life.

Living a life of surrender can be freeing. I will never forget reading about the aftermath of a terrible hurricane. In the calm of the next morning, someone found a straw – a Biblical "slender reed" – lodged into a telephone pole. That straw could never have hoped to do that on its own – it surrendered to the forces that carried it. I imagine myself to be that weak, lifeless straw with no will of its own. I have surrendered not to wind, not to the unfeeling forces of nature or fate, but to God. This helps me live this new life.

Biblical figures

The most Godly people I have known or read about lived their lives this way. They were all in. They didn't just double-down, they shoved all their chips – their strength, their optimism, their will to live – into the middle of the table, and in so doing announced to themselves and the world, "I'm all in." In the Bible, three such men were Elijah, Daniel and Peter.

The prophet Elijah went head-to-head with a false prophet in front of the people. This was a God-sanctioned contest; an ancient reality show. To demonstrate to the people that his God was real, Elijah doused the altar three times with four jars of water before God lit it with fire from heaven in spectacular fashion. Elijah was all in, and was a great man of faith.

Forbidden from worshipping anyone but King Darius, Daniel went ahead and lived his life as though the edict had never been issued:

> When Daniel learnt that this decree had been issued, he went into his house. It had in the roof-chamber windows open towards Jerusalem; and there he knelt down three times a day and offered prayers and praises to his God as was his custom.

That act of faith led to his being thrown into the lion's pit overnight, with a rock covering the opening and sealed with the king's signet "and the signet of his nobles." In the morning, "no wound was found on him, because he had trusted in his God."

And many years later, when Jesus began washing Peter's feet as a way to illustrate humility to the disciples, Peter said something like, "Don't wash my feet! I should be washing your feet!" But Jesus, having the Long View, said, "If I do not wash you, you have no part with me," to which Peter, who was always good at living in the moment, replied, "Then, Lord, not my feet only; wash my hands and head as well!" Peter was all in.

Think of living this new life this way: taking marriage vows is a couple's way of saying "I'm all in." There is no turning back, they are forsaking all others, and they vow to live the rest of their lives loving only that person. For us, there is no turning back. We can only look ahead. We might as well say, "Come what may, I've come this far, I'm all in. Let's do this thing. Let's really live this new life."

What would living "all in" look like?

I propose that living "all in" begins with believing that the hand you have been dealt is not a losing hand at all, nor is it a reason to fold. Losing this high-stakes game we're in, or even playing to a draw, is not an option. If yours is an invisible injury and you look great, nobody can see your cards. And even if they can see your injury, or hear it in your voice, nobody can see your resolve. Your injury, the cards you are holding, can be your secret, and you can wear your poker face, which means you are not letting on to the world that you are disabled.

This chapter opened with some exhortations. Let's look at a few of these more closely and try to apply them with strategies.

Never give up

Never shrink to the dimensions of your disability

Find ways to break the bondage of your injury. Start by freeing yourself from the bondage of somebody else's fear or ignorance. Think about this, and act.

Always fight loneliness and depression

Think about the people who love you truly and deeply. Reach back out to them as they reach out to you. Don't withdraw for longer than short periods. Always come back out in the open and engage with your loved ones. They miss you as much as you miss your old self.

Take time to find pleasure in your new life

Counseling will help you overcome such thoughts as, "I don't deserve to feel good," "I don't deserve to not feel bad," "I don't deserve to heal." This sounds kind of twisted, but look closely at how you feel when you are occasionally able to find pleasure in the midst of your injury. Can you enjoy feeling relatively normal? Now accelerate your self-analysis and ask whether you can permit yourself to enjoy feeling good. If you feel sort of guilty or uncomfortable with even temporary relief from your suffering, professional help sorting through all of that could do wonders for you.

Never apologize to anyone for having a brain injury

If people talk too fast, ask them to repeat what they have said more slowly. Do not apologize for bending the world to your specifications. If you can't answer a question right then and there, say, "That's interesting. Let me think about that one and get back to you."

If your speech or actions make it obvious that you are impaired in some way, even if it's just the time of day and you're tired, you might say something like, "Sometimes I do that. I was in a car accident (or whatever) but I'm working on it." But as far as getting into the details of your injury, never waste your emotional and cognitive resources trying to explain yourself.

Many survivors find that very few people actually want to know what your injury is like anyway, and because it is excruciating to try to explain, especially to someone whose facial expressions you can't read well, save yourself this whole demeaning experience. It usually comes to no good for either of you; if you fail to explain your injury well, neither one of you have found the explanation or even the interaction satisfying. Try saying a few well-practiced phrases, such as, "I've come a long way, and I still have a long road ahead of me, according to my doctor. Thanks for asking." Turn the interaction around, and transition to some other topic that is easier for you.

Practice showing dignity. Be proud that you are a living, breathing human being. Act and speak confidently because you have as much right to the small piece of real estate you are standing on as anyone else. Dare to dream as big as we were intended to dream, and remind yourself who you are. Act and speak as the child of God that you are.

Find ways to be generous in your poverty, grateful in your infirmity

If your injury is more obvious, you can still live your life "all in." None of us can undo what has happened to us, and so we can turn our attentions outward. I believe our lives would look radically different if we lived "as if" we held winning hands. Here's what I mean.

Given that many of us had close brushes with death, in our time remaining – or as some might put it, in the days or years God spared us for – may we be unreasonably generous with our time and our energies and our resources and our talents. May we be kind to everyone we meet. My father once said, "You can tell a person's character by how they treat people they don't need." The more I watch people, the more I see that's true.

Let's ask ourselves, "How can we use who we are to help people in some way? What will be our life's work, both in the short term and the long term? Who can we help right now, even in our condition?"

May we begin each day grateful for another new one, and may our first words never betray our preoccupation: "I" or "I feel" or "I don't feel" or "I'm sorry" or "here's what I need to accomplish today." May we begin simply with thanksgiving for this new day. As the Psalmist says, "Give thanks to the Lord, for he is good; his love endures forever."

To recap: Never give up

LIVING THIS NEW LIFE "AS IF"

The power of the powerless

Although I am a Christian – full disclosure here – I am also an admirer of the work of Christopher Hitchens. He is perhaps best known for his book *God Is Not Great* but long before that I read him eagerly and profitably. His intellect and his wit, it probably goes without saying, are first rate, and he engages me like few other writers and political thinkers.[35]

He makes an intriguing point in his *Letters to a Young Contrarian*, a point that survivors should consider. Recounting his time with dissidents in Eastern Europe in the 1960s, Hitchens writes:

> . . . it was in order to survive . . . that a number of important dissidents evolved a strategy for survival. In a phrase, they decided to live "as if." I'm never certain which author can claim the credit for this mild-sounding but actually deeply subversive and ironic decision. Vaclav Havel . . . called this tactic "The Power of the Powerless" . . . [36]

What if we live our new lives "as if" we are more than just survivors? Does it mean changing our identity, or is it all about rising above our injury – and what does that mean – or is it both, or something else entirely? (I hope these multiple questions did not short-circuit your brain!)

When have you been able to make such a "deeply subversive and ironic decision"? Are you interested? Are you fed up with your life right now? Are all the things you've tried to make your life less miserable working for you? If not, then consider making the deeply subversive and ironic decision to live this new life "as if."

Living this new life as if we were free

Whether or not we are living with a brain injury, we often feel trapped. We always end up face-to-face with our limitations. We are always taught that if we work hard and follow our dream, the sky is the limit. Well, very few people end up flying high in the sky. Henry David Thoreau said, "Most men lead lives of quiet desperation and go to the grave with the song still in them."

I believe that God calls us to freedom. Who are God's people? We are, if we say we are and if we live a life of surrender: "I am Yours. What can You possibly do with this brokenness?" Only in our weakness can God show strength. Only in our bondage can God free us. God led the Israelites out of Egypt and will lead us out of our captivity if we cry out for help; or, as in Job's case, when we pray for our friends ("and the Lord turned Job's captivity when he prayed for his friends").

The phrase "turning captivity" appears not just in Job but in the Psalms, too. This excerpt from Psalm 126 – one of my favorites during my recovery – perfectly captures the intensity of the prayer of desperation, and the plea for freedom and joy:

> When the Lord turned again the captivity of Zion, we were like them that dream.
> Then was our mouth filled with laughter, and our tongue with singing.
> Then said they among the heathen, the Lord hath done great things for them.
> The Lord hath done great things for us, whereof we are glad.
> Turn again our captivity, O Lord, as the streams in the south.
> They that sow in tears shall reap in joy.
> He that goeth forth and weepeth, bearing precious seed shall doubtless come again with rejoicing, bringing his sheaves with him.

I'm grateful that I haven't been taken from my family, but I do feel – every day – that the me that God made has been taken from them and is being worked over and roughed up. Maybe we're broken, but we're not defeated. Maybe we're in captivity, but we can live as though we are free. Maybe we don't know what God has in mind for us and what good will come of our suffering and captivity, but let us be comforted by those words from Jeremiah 29:11:

> For I know the plans I have for you, declares the Lord, plans for wholeness and not for evil, to give you a future and a hope.

Job lost everything, and yet . . .

I'll close with the ubertext on the subject: Job, upon hearing that everything had been taken from him, and his sons and daughters were killed, said:

> Naked I came from the womb; Naked I shall return whence I came. The Lord gives and the Lord takes away; Blessed be the name of the Lord.

Significantly for TBI survivors, Job did not "look great!" Because of the painful sores all over his face and body, Job's friends barely recognized him. His appearance was so extreme that even when they saw him from a distance, they began to weep, and tear their robes, and sprinkle dust on their heads. They came to him and, seeing his great suffering up close and personal, sat on the ground with him for seven days and nights, not saying a word.

What if nobody can see how great your suffering is? I think especially of the veterans coming home from Iraq and Afghanistan, men and women trained to be in great physical shape. Many of them look really great, but their misery is off the charts. I worry about suicide rates among veterans, who have seen and experienced too much, and who feel so alone with their invisible injuries that their new lives are just too much to bear.

We're all chained to this radiator

You might remember the time back in the 1980s when Islamic extremists took hostages in Beirut. After being released, one of the hostages said that before he was kidnapped he did not believe in God. He then began to speak almost wistfully of the endless months he spent handcuffed to a radiator because it was there that he felt God's presence.

The summer evening of one especially bad day, I lay down on the screen porch and closed my eyes to rest before friends came over for dinner. I held a jar of iced tea in one hand, and began to breathe and pray in quiet desperation: "Lord *(inhale)* have *(inhale)* mercy *(inhale)* on *(inhale)* us. Mercy *(inhale)*. Grace *(inhale)*. Peace *(inhale)*. Joy *(inhale)*." I usually found that soothing but in those moments I felt the overwhelming claustrophobia of my injury, and choked up when I prayed, "Lord *(inhale)* save *(inhale)* me!"

The strangest thing happened. My hand suddenly felt the extreme coldness of the jar and I felt that was God's way of saying to me, "I'm here with you." I felt God's closeness with the coldness of the jar. Knowing – fearing – this wouldn't last, but wanting it to, I held on tightly, savoring the sensation.

So my life and perhaps yours has entered a new phase – a life of captivity. We are chained to this radiator, this injury called TBI. May we learn to *turn our captivity*, and experience a kind of freedom that many non-injured people might never know.

May we defy any expectations that we are condemned to a life of depression and withdrawal.

May we surprise ourselves and our loved ones with a newfound generosity of spirit and acts of love.

May we double-down on our new limitations and live this new life "all in," giving away freely what we *do* have.

As for me, if this so-called recovery is any indication of what is ahead, I hope to commune with God as never before. There are times when I have a peace that is beyond understanding. The understanding will have to come later. This is a time for healing.

Afterword

> ". . . so that is all, but it is not enough . . . It is like the man
> who carried a brick with him to show the world what his
> house was like."

Bertolt Brecht

As was true with the video my son Chris made the summer of 2008, this book has aimed at improving the lives of those whose lives have been touched – or hammered – by TBI: survivors, families, friends and professionals.

I set out to give an honest view of what it's like to live with this injury, and compiled a lot of strategies to help survivors get through their new lives in the long-term and each day in the short term.

My friend David suggested in Chapter 6 that the current state of research into the causes of and recovery from a TBI resembles that of AIDS in the early 1980s – there's a serious problem here that is getting away from us, and both the medical community and society is struggling to deal with it. The sheer numbers involved are outstripping anything we have yet come up with to handle the traumatic fallout.

Many chapters in this open up more questions and more possibilities for research and study. Topics for groundbreaking articles and books, both scholarly and for the general reader, that have yet to be written include:

- Minimum common treatments for each unique TBI

- TBI and general nutrition (e.g., Should survivors go easy on carbohydrates? Does data suggest a high-protein diet is beneficial?)

- TBI and nutritional supplements for the body

- TBI and nutritional supplements for the brain (e.g., fish oil, krill oil, CoQ10, a citicoline sodium supplement such as Ceraxon)

- TBI and exercise – cardiovascular and weight-training

- Why do many chemo patients compare their misery with that of brain-injury survivors? What role might Marinol play in relieving our nausea?

- Hyperbaric Oxygen Therapy

- TBI and the baffling chemical world of pharmaceuticals

- TBI and holistic treatments (e.g., acupuncture, yoga, cranial sacral therapy, long outdoor walks)

- TBI and sustaining, even nurturing intimate relationships

Most of you will think of other areas that this book has not addressed. Be assured that more research is being done all the time. More answers and solutions will come. Make your own contributions to the field, as you are able. Be patient. Be strong. Never give up. Always seek out someone if you need help, and be willing to be strong for another survivor who comes to you for support. We need each other. I wish you all the best in your recovery. In fact, I wish you all the best, all the time, forever.

Notes

Notes

Notes

Acknowledgements

I do more than simply acknowledge the contribution and support of these people, I thank them with all my heart:

- Lynne, my heart's desire and the love of my life. I often have dreams in which I'm stuck in a very awkward and increasingly tense situation, and I start looking around for you to come put things right. Is that romantic?

- Our three boys Chris, Andrew and Will, for their love, encouragement, understanding and many acts of kindness.

- Laura Ricard, without whose brain, energy and enthusiasm I could not have completed this book.

- Survivors whose stories appear in the book. This book is our story.

- Marrilee Wilson, Michelle Domey and Elizabeth Thyng Montanaro, for their friendship as evidenced by their emails, texts, and phonecalls, all of which serve to lighten my burden in so many ways – not least of which is making me laugh and hearing them laugh.

- My friends in the Amazing Brain Injury Survivor Support Group of Framingham, MA.

- The incredible medical professionals at Spaulding Rehabilitation Hospital in Boston, and the Brain Injury Research Center at Mount Sinai Medical Center in NYC.

- Marilyn Spivack, founder of the BIA over 30 years ago, for her strong encouragement to write this book in the first place.

- Madelaine Sayko, brain-injury advocate, educator, and now friend, for her insight and energy, not to mention her thoughtful inquiries into my well-being. Her urging me never to give up has helped me to press on in this important work.

- Pastor Michael Hintze and the congregation of Our Savior Lutheran Church, Westminster MA for their many examples of saintliness.

- Joshua Caleb Weibley, for creating the artwork on the cover of both the DVD and this book. ("Mom, it's my profile. How about if I hold it out like this?")

- Mike Maginn, President and CEO of Singularity Group, for helping to facilitate a "best practices" session at one of our support-group meetings in Framingham, MA. He has taken an avid interest not only in my recovery, but in exploring ways of enhancing the lives of the brain-injured.

Recovery Team

Of all the members of my recovery team, I must first give a loud shout-out to my friend and recovery mentor Rick Sanders (M.S. CCC-SLP, M.T.S.), my SLP at Spaulding Rehabilitation Hospital in Boston. As you've seen throughout this book, Rick made many valuable comments to the manuscript. Beyond that, however, he has been a model for me on how to 1) listen to survivors with greater empathy and sensitivity, and 2) be a more compassionate, more selfless human being.

Speech-Language Pathologists everywhere would do well to emulate Rick. Year after year, he teaches graduate students that they must learn about TBI from their patients, and not *only* from the requisite medical literature.

Other members of my recovery team include, but are not limited to (in alphabetical order):

- **Beth Adams**, Licensed Rehabilitation Counselor (M. Ed. LRC)

- **Sally Johnson**, MSW, LICSW

- **Jason Krellman**, Ph.D.; NYS Licensed Psychologist; Post-Doctoral Fellow in Rehabilitation Research and Clinical Neuropsychology, Department of Rehabilitation Medicine, Mount Sinai School of Medicine (when I worked with him)

- **Kaloyan S. Tanev**, M.D., Director of Clinical Neuropsychiatry Research at Massachusetts General Hospital

- **Ross Zafonte**, D.O, Vice President of Medical Affairs and Chair of the Department of Physical Medicine and Rehabilitation (PMR) at Harvard Medical School; Vice President of Medical Affairs for Spaulding Rehabilitation Hospital Boston, MA

My team has greatly enriched me with their wisdom, and both their professional and personal attentions. I am very grateful to each of them.

Readers

Finally, many thanks to my insightful and selfless readers, who let me borrow their brains for awhile. I knew I could turn to them for incisive commentary, and they came through for me big time:

- Readers of pertinent chapters: Rick Sanders, Sally Johnson and Beth Adams

- Readers of early drafts: Ann Hintze and Dorothy Yep

- Readers of almost final drafts: Andrew Byler; Chris Byler; Timothy J. "misplaced modifier" Bleecker, Ph.D.; Bob MacDonald; Lynne and Will Byler; and Elizabeth Tuttle (my favorite Fulbright Scholar)

- Reader of what I thought was final draft: Hannah V. Hintze, Ph.D. (my favorite classical scholar and an all 'round mensch)

APPENDICES

APPENDIX A:

Feedback on Video:

"You Look Great!" – Inside a Traumatic Brain Injury

APPENDIX B:

Audience for This Book

APPENDIX C:

The Prevalence and Toll of TBI

APPENDIX D:

"Blast Injury and TBI" *(excerpt)*

APPENDIX E:

Tips for Getting through an MRI

APPENDIX F:

Q&A with Mike about the TBI/Endocrinology Connection

APPENDIX A – Feedback on Video:
"You Look Great!" – Inside a Traumatic Brain Injury

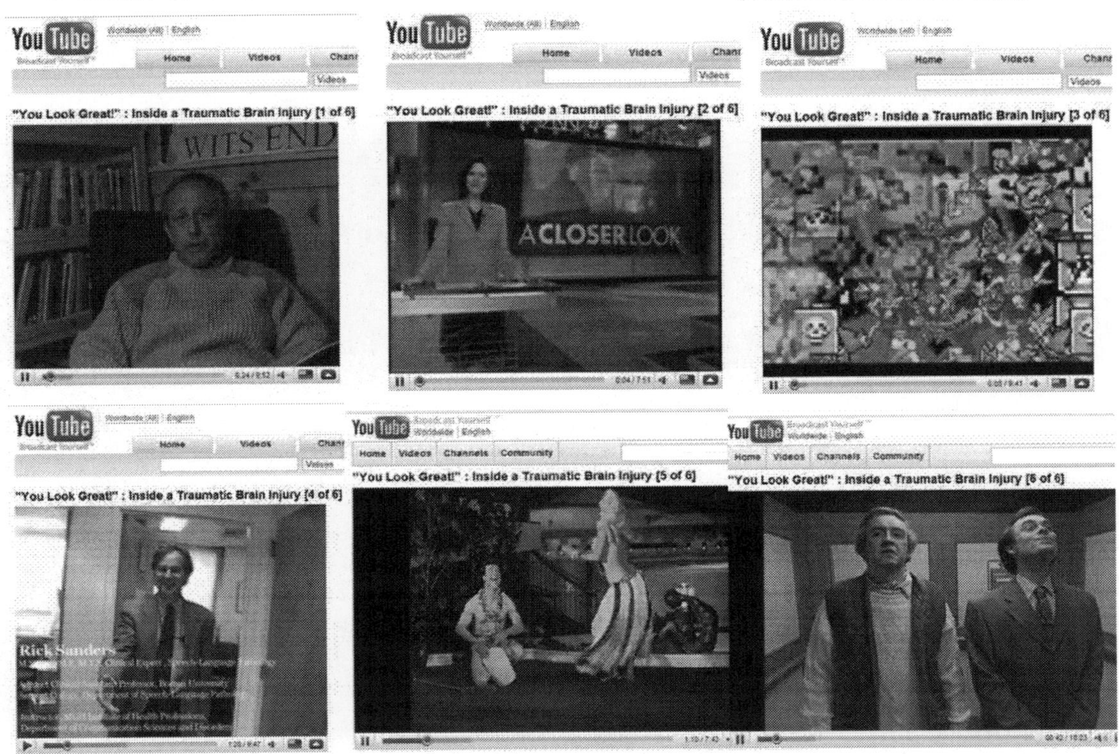

This short film is a must-see for anyone whose life touches mild TBI: survivors, families, friends, and professionals. With great insight, courage and humor, John gives us a rare view of what it's like to live with this injury. His story, images, and metaphors open up a world typically closed, invisible, ignored, or misunderstood.

Marilyn Spivack, founder of the Brain Injury Association of America

```
Great inspirational video! Well told, I love the media
incorporated throughout. Just added you to our playlist of
must watch TBI videos.
```

Brainline.org

I took a look at the videos, and I LOVED them. Thanks so much for sharing these! They are going to be SUCH a good resource for our TBI warriors, who took often feel a bit overlooked. Thanks!

Wounded Warrior Project

I think this is such a great tool. May I share it with my friends and family? It is hard for them to see the impact. This would help.

Outstanding! You've touched on every issue I've experienced since experiencing my mTBI from a rear end collision . . . Your work brings clarity to a difficult to explain topic.

I'm so glad to have found this wonderful set of videos. *Thank you* for all the effort it took to put them together. Thanks for the story, the laughs, and the renewed hope.

I've been dealing with TBI aftermath for 19 years. Your presentation touched on every aspect and has been a comfort. Thank you for your bravery and effort in putting this together.

This was a great set of videos. I am a children's nurse in England working in a rehab unit for children with ABI and TBI. I found your story very insightful and engaging. Cheers and good luck in the future!

Your videos are much more than useful. You describe the blueprint of a substantial portion of my TBI in a way that I am unable to articulate even though I understand the difficulty.   :-)

I keep saying to my husband that is just like me. Your description of the "Catch 22" problem was spot on!!! So many thanks for all of this effort. Seems overwhelming to me. Thanks for speaking for all of us.

Thanks so much for putting this together. You have told my story as you tell yours. So hard for others to get inside our head. "How are you?" that was always a hard one.

Congratulations John!! You and your son have done an amazing job on this. It is sure to help many survivors and family members, and provide insights for healthcare professionals. Congratulations again.

Your videos are remarkable . . . and help provide a view into the unknown. I am a caregiver for my wife and it is hard for her to communicate to me what is going on. Thank you and please keep up the good work. I have gotten a lot out of it. I would like to think that other caregivers would too.

(My wife) watched about half of all your videos, but the look on her face was awesome like she was relating and concentrating. She doesn't do that too much any other time. When something caught her attention, she perked up and squinted her eyes to watch.

Thank you for recording this series. I have posted all six of your videos on Facebook and began posting one at a time on my MySpace. I hope you will continue recording videos, as you proceed on your journey. We need them. I further appreciated that your videos did not focus predominantly on our troops. Not that I want to diminish their injuries. My concern in that aspect is, that with so much focus on services for our troops who have sustained TBI's, the rest of us might slip through the cracks.

Wonderful presentation!! I wrote (down) a few of your priceless phrases like "residual intelligence".

The language you used to express what it's like on the inside of a TBI was amazing to say the least. Even a layperson can grasp the essential elements of a TBI, as you simplify what in my mind at least seems to be so complicated.

Stumbling blindly through the ambiguous haze of TBI for a decade . . . I am no longer able to work. It's gotten harder to effectively clarify the difficulties and that is where your videos, for me, have been most helpful. Thank you!

Thank you, thank you, thank you. I cannot thank you enough. Your video is a revelation. . . . You must get it distributed professionally. You articulate and express information regarding TBI that no one else has. Again, I would like to reiterate what a revelation your videotape is.

I just wanted to say, thank you for taking the time to put up your videos to help those of us trying to understand more about TBI and its effects. I need to know all I can about it and the long-term effects. Thank you so much for sharing and may God bless you always.

Thanks so much. You put into words and images what I am going through. I struggle to explain this to people but am unable to. I look great. I even worked for the first two months, trudging on in a fog, suffering from horrible headaches and a host of other symptoms. I was told by a neurologist right after the accident that whatever symptoms remained at 3 months would be permanent and there was nothing I could do, that I didn't need a follow up. Ultimately I got worse and got help. Thanks.

Thank you so much for making this video. I sustained a TBI in August of 09 due to being hit by a careless driver. I'm fortunate in some ways; my MRIs, CAT scans and EEGs confirmed the diagnosis of TBI. I have difficulty putting into words what it's like now living with a TBI. I watched your video and cried, knowing I wasn't alone. My family now has a better understanding of what my TBI is like for me. Again, thank you.

Thanks to you and Chris for putting together such great videos! Watching them was almost like someone putting everything I feel and deal with into words and pictures! Thank you! I hope you don't mind I will be sharing them! Thanks for your resources at the end as well as sharing your experience and helping others like myself feel not so alone!

Chris and I entered a 6-minute version of the video in the 2011 Neuro Film Festival. Just before going to print with this revised edition of the book, the good people behind Doonesbury selected it for its daily selection. The first four seconds condense the entire 55-minute original film, and then moves on to make the case for contributing to brain injury research.

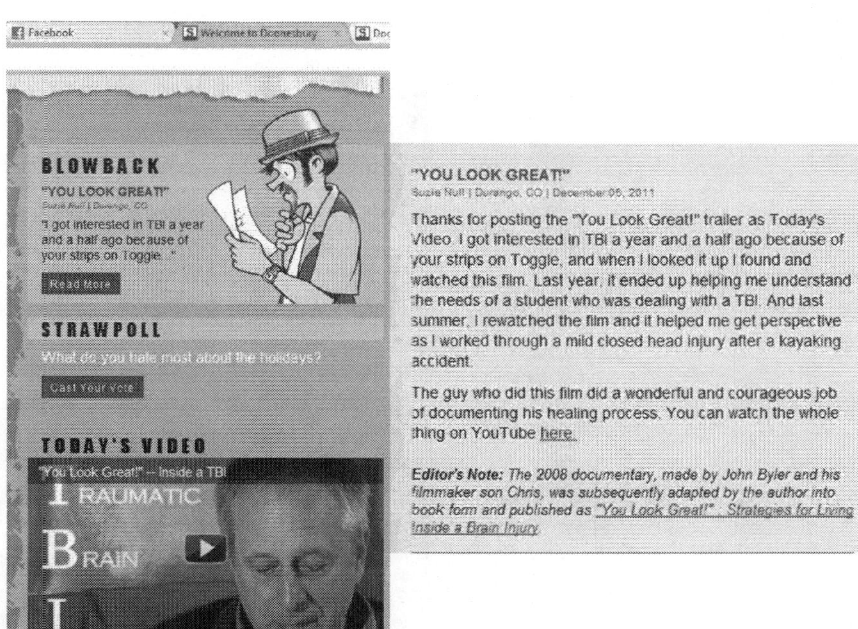

APPENDIX B – Audience for this Book

<u>Primary audience</u>: TBI survivors and their caregivers, families, and friends

Primarily, this book is for:

- Survivors of a traumatic brain injury – "mild" or otherwise – who are desperate for practical and professional guidance, and assurance that what they are going through is not unusual for someone with this injury; there is strength in numbers, and they are not alone

- Family, friends, and caregivers of TBI survivors who want insight into their loved one's experience

Someone with a brain injury, as well as their loved ones and caretakers, face a baffling amount of information and misinformation, often from professionals, and no good way to sort through it all. They crave a straightforward explanation of what has just happened, what to expect next, and how to make a bad situation more tolerable.

This book tells how survivors, their loved ones and their caregivers can begin navigating the complicated and difficult task of recovery. People recovering from a stroke have said, "This is my story, too," as have brain surgery patients and even cancer patients undergoing chemotherapy who often experience what they call "chemo brain."

<u>Secondary audience</u>: Medical professionals, neurolawyers, therapists, counselors, medical students

This book will help medical professionals of every stripe answer these

questions:

- "Does my patient have a traumatic brain injury?"

- "What do I currently use as criteria for even a preliminary diagnosis of a brain injury?"

- "What are some clear indicators of a TBI, beyond the physical evidence of a CT scan and MRI?"

- "What is my patient going through? What is day-to-day life like?"

- "What medical professionals should I be referring this patient to?"

- "What role, if any, does psychiatric analysis play in sorting out the patient's mental health as distinct from what might be a brain injury?"

TBI and recovery from same will continue to be better understood, and the

next generation of professionals needs to be well-prepared. This book provides

guidance in recognizing TBI symptoms and how to determine as soon as

possible an accurate diagnosis and the best course for recovery.

Therefore, this book is also for:

- Medical professionals who need a close look at life inside of a TBI, such as, but not limited to, neurologists, endocrinologists, neuropsychiatrists, neuropsychologists, and psychopharmacologists (each of whom can play a crucial role in your recovery, which I explain);

- Other medical professionals who must learn to recognize symptoms of a TBI, including, but certainly not limited to, EMT first-responders, Attending Physicians in Emergency Rooms, general practitioners, and pediatricians;

- Professionals who need a close look at life inside of a TBI, such as – but not limited to – neurotrauma rehabilitation counselors, Case Managers, neurolawyers, social workers, Speech Language Pathologists (SLP), and vocational rehabilitation counselors;

- Psychologists and psychiatrists for two important reasons: 1) Although they cannot promise healing from a TBI, they can help survivors improve the quality of their lives, creating a healthier mental environment in which to heal; and 2) TBI – especially mild TBI – is often misdiagnosed as mental illness or simple lack of motivation to get better;

- Students who are preparing to enter any of the above professions, and who need to go beyond textbook case-study accounts to understand the effects of TBI and strategies for recovery.

APPENDIX C – The Prevalence and Toll of TBI

TRAUMATIC STATISTICS!

Each year, there are more Traumatic Brain Injuries than new cases of multiple sclerosis, spinal cord injuries, HIV/AIDS, and breast cancer – combined. This lists those who have merely been _diagnosed_ in the U.S. with a traumatic brain injury _annually_.

- Traumatic brain injuries: 1,700,000

- Breast cancer: 205,000

- HIV/AIDS: 41,289

- Spinal cord injuries: 11,000

- Multiple sclerosis: 10,400

Source: Center on Brain Injury Research and Training (CBIRT.org/resources)

The Center for Disease Control and Prevention (CDC) has increased the estimate to 1.7 million people who sustain a TBI annually, and of those 1.7 million:

- 52,000 die,

- 275,000 are hospitalized

- 1,365,000 emergency department visits; nearly 80% are treated and released

Consider the wealth of resources and public awareness of many of the other injuries and diseases listed above, and then try to recall the last time you were asked to contribute money for research on healing and recovery from a traumatic brain injury. Clearly, given the prevalence and devastation of the injury, TBI is under-represented in all kinds of ways, including diagnosis, treatment, research, and fund-raising efforts.

Now consider these figures:

- TBI is a contributing factor to a third (30.5%) of all injury-related deaths in the United States

- About 75% of TBIs that occur each year are concussions or other forms of mild TBI

<u>Source</u>: Center for Disease Control and Prevention

Note that only 25% of TBIs, therefore, are severe cases.

Consider too the drain on America's economy:

- Brain injuries require 3.5 million days of hospitalization and loss of more than 35,000 years of productive work annually

- Hospital and facilities costs relating to TBI in the U.S. is estimated to **exceed $48 billion annually**

<u>Source</u>: Brain Injury Association of Massachusetts

As I've mentioned, TBI is chronically misdiagnosed and under-diagnosed, a fact which tells us that the numbers quoted above are conservative estimates. Also, these statistics tell us how prevalent the injury is in the U.S., but of course TBI is not exclusively an American phenomenon. And if these numbers under-represent the U.S., how much greater is the risk for brain injury in countries without the benefit of U.S. safety regulations and medical facilities.

WHO IS AT RISK FOR A TBI?

According to the Brain Injury Association of Massachusetts, the most common causes of brain injury are:

- Motor vehicle accidents (by far)

- Falls

- Violence and handguns

- Sport and recreational accidents

- Work-related accidents

I'll review just a few groups here:

Roughly one-fifth of our returning Armed Forces

It is often said that TBI has become the signature injury of the Iraq war. When an improvised exploding device – an IED – blasts, if you survive it, your brain is violently shaken inside the skull. (*See Appendix C: "Blast Injury and TBI"*)

So think about all those soldiers coming home with traumatic brain injuries. Maybe they have all four limbs and maybe not, but those soldiers could suffer neurotrauma for years – or for the rest of their lives. This is because sometimes the neurons heal, and sometimes they don't; often, if the brain does heal, it heals very . . . very . . . slowly.

Anyone active in sports at any level of competition

The CDC estimates that "Nearly one in every ten athletes who play contact sports suffers a concussion or mild brain injury *each season*. More than 60,000

sports-related concussions occur annually in high school contact sports."
(underline and italics mine)

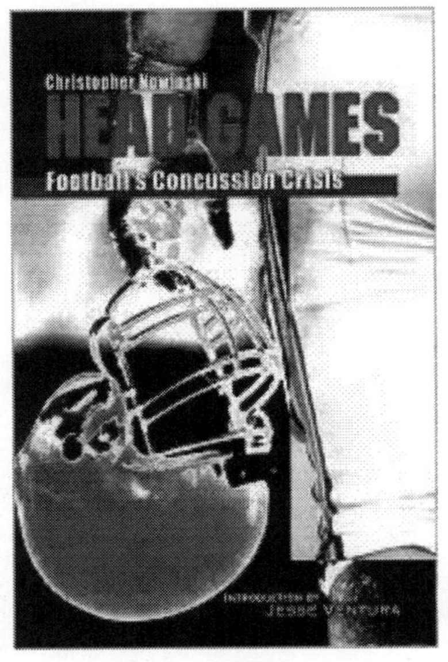

I recommend Christopher Nowinski's 2006 book, *Head Games: Football's Concussion Crisis from the NFL to the Youth Leagues*. Chris played football at Harvard and became the two-time, youngest ever World Wrestling Entertainment Hardcore Champion. In his public speaking and in his book, he doesn't say kids shouldn't play sports or that football players should start playing touch football.

Citing his own excellent research he poses the critical question:

> Who should be the one telling an athlete at any level –from Little League to high school to the pros – when or even whether to get back in the game?

The coach? He might say or imply, "Suck it up, kid. We need you."

The trainer? Have they been educated in the signs of neurotrauma?

The player? Not to state the bleeding obvious but if you've just suffered a concussion your judgment is impaired and you don't make good decisions. "I'm fine! I just want to play, coach!"

The parent, or even the athlete's personal physician?

Chris points out quite frankly that these people, as well intentioned as they might be, do not know enough about the brain and its capacity for injury to make that decision.

To further spotlight TBI, the *New York Times'* Alan Schwartz has written some excellent articles on concussion in the NFL and high schools, and its devastating effects on current and retired players.

Besides football and soccer, concussions are common in other sports too. Giving a guy a concussion is the whole point of boxing, and who should tell a boxer to get up off the stool and answer the bell? The spit-bucket guy? Don King?

Next to Ultimate Fighting, boxing is considered almost genteel. Ultimate Fighting is a hugely popular sport that involves repeated blows to the head using knees, feet, elbows and fists.

And remember the old joke, "I went to a boxing match and a hockey game broke out"?

Now think of the role sports plays in America . . . at the elementary school, high school, college, and of course professional levels. How many times will a totally buff athlete hear the words, "You look great!" with the possible subtext of, "Why aren't you on the field?" (Go to sportsconcussion.net/ for more information.)

And those of us in the business world can sense or even hear the same thing. If we can occasionally manage a friendly, informal lunch or dinner with a former colleague, a facial expression or outright question might be, "So . . . why aren't you back at work?" Again, TBI can be an invisible injury.

Anyone who rides in a motor vehicle

I read about a woman who was hit from behind in her car at a stop sign by a car going only 15 mph. She seemed fine at the time. At that speed she basically just felt a sharp nudge. Over the next week though, her body and her brain gradually absorbed the shock. She suffered a devastating brain injury, called "mild" because it was not more severe and she looked fine.

At one of my presentations I asked, "How many of you are in the NFL?" No hands went up. "How many of you are professional wrestlers?" No hands. "How many of you have just returned from Iraq?" No hands. "How many of you got here in a car?" All hands went up.

APPENDIX D – "Blast Injury and TBI" *(excerpt)*

by Ronald C. Savage, EdD, Executive Vice President, North American Brain Injury Society (NABIS)

The war in Iraq will be no different in producing a "signature wound" only this time the wound is in the brains of those affected. Medical experts are witnessing an emerging and significant increase in Traumatic Brain Injury (TBI). In other words, the Iraq war could produce a generation of veterans with life changing brain injury, affecting thousands of service men and women from all walks of life across the country.

During the Vietnam War and the Persian Gulf War, 76 percent of American troops survived combat wounds. But in this century, the U.S. military's surgical teams "have saved the lives of an unprecedented 90 percent of the soldiers wounded in battle…" (*New England Journal of Medicine*, December, 2006). Furthermore, Walter Reed Army Medical Center reported that nearly 30% of all patients with combat-related injuries seen at Walter Reed from 2003 to 2005 sustained a TBI and that blast injuries are a significant cause of TBIs. In addition, they reported that TBI is often associated with severe multiple trauma, post traumatic stress disorder (PTSD) or undiagnosed concussions. Thus, screening soldiers who are at risk for a TBI is important in order to ensure that TBIs are identified and appropriately treated.

Diagnosis can be difficult even when TBI is apparent or the patient is able to describe a concussive head injury to their doctors. The more common mild brain injury often has more than mild consequences and can cause depression, reduced cognitive functioning, nausea, sleep disturbance, erratic behavior, and mood swings. These impairments are exacerbated by misdiagnosis, lack of treatment and the public's misperceptions about brain injury and mental illness. For veterans with brain injuries, the lack of physical signs and the diffuse nature of symptoms may be met with skepticism, considered to be psychological, or worse, malingering.

As professionals in the field know, the "walking wounded" do not disappear. And many more will be seen and heard in this decade. Thanks to improvements in protective gear and swift medical treatment, more of America's wounded are surviving - and returning home with serious, permanent injuries. How will these veterans fare in the routines of daily life? Will they be able to maintain employment? How will their injuries impact their families, friends, co-workers, and communities?

The North American Brain Injury Society has begun to address these important issues.

APPENDIX E – Tips for Getting through an MRI

Here's what helps you spend 30 to 40 minutes inside the coffin of the MRI.

If you think you will be claustrophobic, it's common to be prescribed Valium, which will take the edge off your anxiety.

Lie down and the technician will give you a rubber thing you can squeeze once you're inside in case you panic and need to come out. You'll hold that on your chest. Place your other hand on your thigh. This helps ground you in a way, to let your body know that you're not totally inside.

Then close your eyes, because the technician will close a metal cage around your face. Looking at it might increase your sense of claustrophobia.

Keep your eyes closed as you feel the platform you're on moving. Keep them closed until you come out. Now you're going to have to find a way to pass the time.

This is the most important part: With your free hand on your thigh, tap each finger to go along with a word to something. I did this for The Lord's Prayer because I knew I would remember all the words. So it would go like this:

> **Our** (tap pinky) **Father** (tap ring finger), **who** (tap middle finger) **art** (tap index finger) **in** (tap thumb) **Heaven** (tap pinky), **hallowed** (tap ring finger) **be** (tap middle finger) **Thy** (tap index finger) **name** (tap thumb).

I also tried doing this for the 23rd Psalm – "The Lord is my shepherd," and so on – but I couldn't remember all the words. This actually turned out fine because I would go as far as I remembered and just start over again, which distracted me from my confinement.

Of course, you can also use this method with any old song; for example the Allman Brothers' "Whipping Post":

> **I've** (tap pinky) **been** (tap ring finger) **run** (tap middle finger) **down** (tap index finger), **I've** (tap thumb) **been** (tap pinky) **lied** (tap ring finger) **to** (tap middle finger). **I** (tap index finger) **don't** (tap thumb) **know** (tap pinky) **why** (tap ring finger) **I** (tap middle finger) **let** (tap index finger) **that** (tap thumb) **mean** (tap pinky) **woman** (tap ring finger) **make** (tap middle finger) **me** (tap index finger) **a fool** (tap thumb).

By the way, you'll hear loud knocking sounds, like you're under the hood of a car that's running on really bad gasoline. Pay it no mind. Just keep tapping your fingers.

The only other thing you might hear is the technician asking you if you're all right. Don't open your eyes. Just say you're fine. You'll be out of there in no time. In fact, as she rolled me out I was feeling pretty cocky – maybe it was the Valium – and I thought I could stay in there longer.

APPENDIX F – Q&A with Mike about the TBI/Endocrinology Connection

<u>Question:</u> Why did you think you might have an endocrinology problem?

<u>Answer:</u> I read that TBI can cause hypopituitarism. What happened was, one of the immediate things I had a problem with I noticed after injury was almost total loss of libido. So at some point, probably six months or so after they determined I had TBI, my GP checked my testosterone level. There are different tables, but what they do is they give you a range that's normal. For men ages 18 to 65 it's a big range, a wide spectrum. They fall into a range between 200-1100. Mine was measured the first time and several times after extremely low, way below 200. What happened was, my PCP initially treated it with testosterone replacement therapy, a gel that you rub on your skin. I stayed on that for close to a year, and the level just wasn't increasing. It was an insignificant increase and wasn't working for me.

So my doctor wanted me to have an endocrinology workup, which I had done at [a highly respected hospital]. When I met with the neuroendocrinologist, he told me he had participated in a study having to do with hormonal deficiencies and TBI, and learned that growth hormone is usually the first to go.

So I had bloodwork done, which showed low testosterone, problems with ACTH, another hormone, and a very low IGF 1. How they initially look at growth hormone, and they dialed down into further tests called stimulation tests, and what they do is, I had a growth hormone stimulation test done, they actually put growth hormone releasing agents into you, a two-hour long test, to measure whether or not pituitary gland has ability to produce hormones.

What was tough was that I had several interactions with the doctor who told me I was deficient in human growth hormone, and my test results confirmed that, and how much would help me and then the doctor says no to me over the phone.

At that point I started to look for specialists who dealt with endocrinology and TBI. I found a lot of information about it online and evidently it's a lot more common for people to have endocrinology problems after TBI. Studies indicate that 40% of people with TBI have some type of endocrinology problem. I was recommended two specialists, not in TBI, but in pituitary-specific problems. I contacted both of them, in another part of the country.

Question: What were the benefits after all of that?

Answer: The first appointment I had a lot of testing out there and he determined that I had hypopituitariasm. They prescribed intermuscular injections for testosterone, which brought my level back to where it should be.

The testosterone corrected my libido and energy levels. I'd worked out with weights in a gym prior to the injury and I was unable to before getting my hormones corrected. It helped my speech, which was much worse than it is now, and helped with making eye contact, my overall mood, and a general sense of well being. I was more or less comatose before I got onto the hormone replacement therapy.

The doctor explained that typically there are two glands in the brain, the pituitary and behind it is the hypothalamus, and the latter controls the pituitary. They are connected by microscopic axons just like the gray matter in the brain. And his thought was, although I presented as having hypopituitariasm, that what probably caused it was the tearing of the neurons or axons between the hypothalamus and the pituitary. That is a big issue because stimulation tests are simply seeing whether the pituitary has the ability to produce a hormone. And that's a problem, because the pituitary could produce growth hormone under stimulation, if the connection is disrupted. Although the pituitary operates under stimulation, it will never operate on its own correctly.

I take testosterone by way of intermuscular injection, which is an at-home treatment. I inject the testosterone into my buttocks with a two-inch needle.

I take the HCG twice a week. The needle is a half-inch, about the size of what a diabetic uses. I inject that into my abdomen at bedtime. I can do that one on my own if I have to.

Question: How important do you think it is for a TBI survivor to have a complete endocrinology work-up?

Answer: It's definitely critical to have an endocrinologist on the recovery team, to have your hormones checked. And from there on, if there's a problem to involve an endocrinologist. Why that isn't done immediately is what's puzzling to me, since it's present 40% of people with TBI, why isn't it protocol to do it right away.

Index

Adams, Beth (*see also: case manager*) 45, 115, 123, 163, 164

About the Authors

John C. Byler

John lives in Harvard, MA with his wife Lynne and, when they come home to visit, their all grown-up and moved-out sons Chris, Andrew and Will. He will forever be grateful for their unconditional love, their lifelines of support and their often random but healing senses of humor. John serves on the Board of the Brain Injury Association of Massachusetts (BIA-MA), and on the Cross-Disability Advisory Council at Boston's Disability Law Center. He enjoys things that he likes. Shout out to his mother Bonnie Scheid and to his friends.

Laura Ricard, Ph.D.

Although John tried several attempts at drafting an elaborate, fairly witty bio for Laura Ricard, Ph.D., she maintains that she is simply a professional writer who lives in Amherst, MA. (She is much more than that, though. Trust me.)

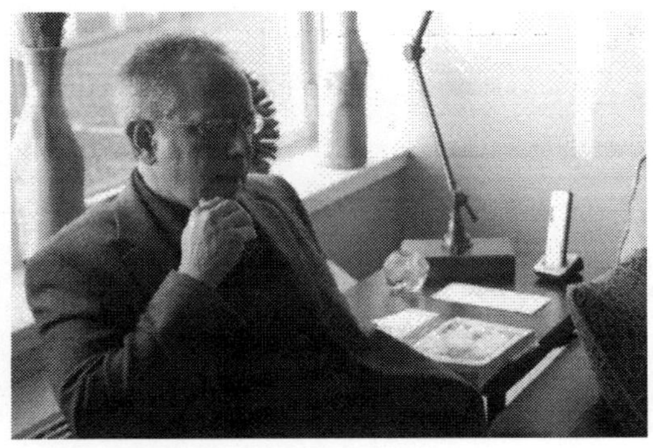

John in full flight, explaining the finer points of finding a good case manager, or more likely expanding on the topic of why lunch was so great

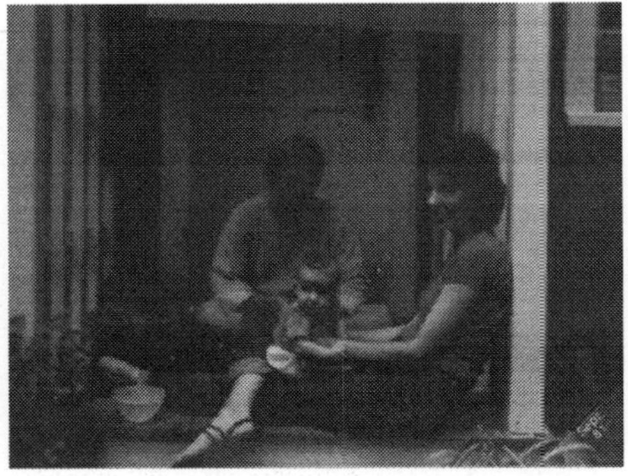

(9/1981) John, his sister-in-law Laura Ricard and her daughter Sarah, who now dances with the Pacific Northwest Ballet. Her son Noel'le Longhaul studies printmaking at RISD.

About John's Grandmother, Edna Ruth Byler, no stranger to beating the odds

Edna Ruth Byler, born 22 May 1904, was the daughter of Benjamin Miller and Anna May Weaver and grew up near Hesston, Kansas. She attended a one-room school, and a Mennonite church made up mostly of Pennsylvania Dutch people. She graduated from Hesston College in 1923. While at the college, Professor J. N. Byler (d. 14 February 1962) noticed her, and they were married in 1925. He was 30, she was 21. By 1928 they had their first child, Donna Lou. Delmar was born in 1930.

In 1939 they moved to Boulder, Colorado, where J. N. Byler pursued a Ph.D. degree. They returned to Hesston in 1941, then traveled to the East, where Mennonite Central Committee (MCC) administrators asked J. N. Byler to oversee what eventually became relief work in unoccupied France. Edna stayed behind with the two children and became housemother for the unit workers at MCC headquarters in Akron, Pennsylvania. When her husband returned in 1942, the workers were calling her "Mrs. B."

On a trip to Puerto Rico with her husband, Edna saw the needlework of poor women and agreed to market it. With crafts added later, this became the MCC SELFHELP Crafts program (later Ten Thousand Villages). She also operated a gift shop until her death on 6 July 1976.

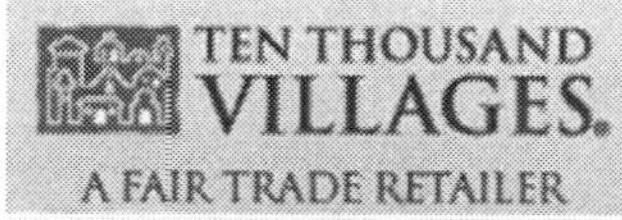

OUR HISTORY

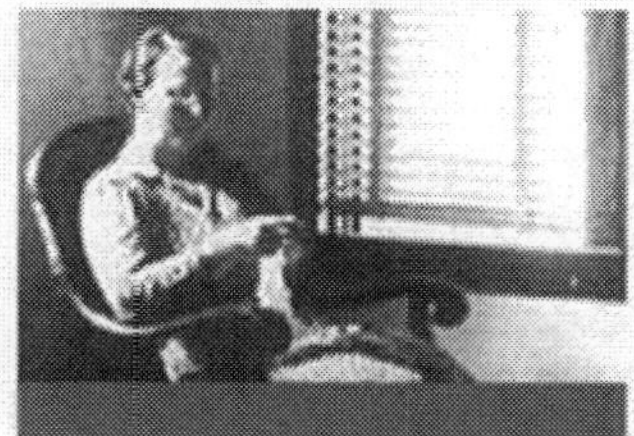

The global fair trade movement began with the founding of Ten Thousand Villages more than 60 years ago through the visionary work of Edna Ruth Byler, a pioneering businesswoman. Byler was struck by the overwhelming poverty she witnessed during a trip to Puerto Rico in 1946, where she was moved to take action. The seminal contribution of Byler ignited a global movement to eradicate poverty through market-based solutions.

Byler believed that she could provide sustainable economic opportunities for artisans in developing countries by creating a viable marketplace for their products in North America. She began a grassroots campaign among her family and friends in the United States by selling handcrafted products out of the trunk of her car. Byler made a concerted effort to educate her community about the lives of artisans around the world.

For the next 30 years, Byler worked tirelessly to connect individual entrepreneurs in developing countries with market opportunities in North America. From humble beginnings, Ten Thousand Villages has grown to a global network of social entrepreneurs working to empower and provide economic opportunities to artisans in developing countries.

Endnotes

[1] www.cdc.gov/TraumaticBrainInjury/statistics.html

[2] A couple of times during a presentation, I paused after I said this, looked at the audience and said, "like a tuneless, malodorous accordion." Nobody ever laughed so I stopped saying it. For the same reason I stopped saying at the very beginning, "Thank you for having me here tonight. I will remember our time together for the rest of the day."

[3] "Coping With Uncertainty After Injury to the Brain," *New York Times*, July 3, 2007

[4] www.biama.org/docs/sportsfacts.doc

[5] "The Daily Checkup: Unclouding the mysteries of the mind," by Katie Charles, *Daily News*, Tuesday, March 25th 2008

[6] Mt Sinai Hospital Traumatic Brain Injury (TBI) Central

[7] Dr. Joe Congeni, You Tube; "Concussions Can Have Delayed Consequences"; WLWT-TV Cincinnati

[8] "The Tragic Death of Natasha Richardson," May/June 2009, *Neurology Now*, quoting Rolland S. Parker, PhD, a neuropsychologist in private practice in New York City, and adjunct professor of clinical neurology at NYU School of Medicine.

[9] *Webster's Third International Dictionary*

[10] Both Ed Harris and Gary Oldman have played Beeethoven in the movies. They also starred together in "State of Grace" with Sean Penn, who has yet to portray the great composer.

[11] Formerly the Joint Commission on Accreditation of Healthcare Organizations (JCAHO)

[12] www.endotext.org/neuroendo12

[13] Ibid

[14] For more information, visit the Hormone Foundation website at www.hormone.org. See also, "What is an Endocrinologist?" at www.hormone.org/public/endocrinologist.cfm

[15] Neurotrauma Registry: http://neurotraumaregistry.com

[16] Ibid

[17] Copyright ©1999, 2000, 2001 Dennis P. Swiercinsky, Ph.D
http://www.brainsource.com/nptests.htm   Note that 67 tests were listed on this website

[18] To get a general idea of what neuropsychological tests measure, and how many kinds of tests exist, you might want to check out Swiercinsky's website: www.brainsource.com/nptests.htm

[19] The Patient tab at www.nora.cc

[20] Ibid

[21] www.ascpp.org

[22] Ibid

[23] Quoting Liat Ayalon, PhD, with the University of California, San Diego, in "Mild Head Injuries Increase Risk of Sleep Disorders," *ScienceDaily*, April 3, 2007, citing a study published in the April 3, 2007, issue of *Neurology*, the scientific journal of the American Academy of Neurology

[24] "Brain Injuries May Result in Trouble Sleeping, Study Finds," *ScienceDaily*, May 25, 2010, citing a study published in the May 25, 2010, issue of *Neurology.*

[25] "Treating Sleep Disorders In People With Traumatic Brain Injury May Not Eliminate Symptoms," *ScienceDaily*, April 15, 2009

[26] Ibid

[27] "Imbalance following traumatic brain injury in adults: Causes and characteristics," *Neurology Report*, March 1999 by Leslie Allison

[28] "Blast Induced Traumatic Brain Injury and Vestibular Pathology in US Military," APTA, 2009-10-16. (Read more at: www.disabled-world.com/health/neurology/tbi/)

[29] Robert T. Fraser, Ph.D., CRC, Paul Wehman, Ph.D., Pamela Targett, M.Ed., *Employment Strategies and Resources* (Harbinger Press, 2010)

[30] Visit his website at www.kolpan.com to learn more about the many benefits of hiring a good brain injury lawyer.

---

[31] Zafonte is the Earle P. and Ida S. Charlton Professor and Chairman of the Department of Physical Medicine and Rehabilitation at Harvard Medical School. His research has been funded by the National Institute of Health and the National Institute on Disability and Rehabilitation Research, as well as the Department of Defense. In 2006, Dr. Zafonte received the Walter Zeiter Award and Lectureship by the American Academy of Physical Medicine and Rehabilitation, and in 2008 he received the Association of Academic Physiatrists' Distinguished Academician Award. He is consistently on the *List of America's Top Doctors* and *Best Doctors in America*.

[32] R. Richard Sanders, M.S. CCC-SLP, M.T.S.; Certificate of Clinical Competence, American Speech-Language-Hearing Association, current since 1980; Massachusetts Licensed Speech-Language Pathologist, current since 1984

[33] Dr. Gordon is the Jack Nash Professor of Rehabilitation Medicine and an Associate Director of the Department of Rehabilitation Medicine at Mount Sinai School of Medicine. He is also Chief of the Rehabilitation Psychology and Neuropsychology service. Dr. Gordon is a Diplomate in Clinical Neuropsychology and a Fellow in the Academy of Behavioral Medicine Research. He provides diagnostic (neuropsychological evaluation) and treatment (psychotherapy, cognitive remediation) for individuals who have sustained a brain injury from trauma, a medical event or exposure to toxic substances, such as mold.

[34] Rick Sanders agrees: "Some people have benefited greatly from using a digital or sports watch of the kind made by Casio and Timex. You can set numerous types of alarms including a beep on the hour or a specific hour or a countdown timer to beep after a certain amount of elapsed time. You can also use your cell phone to do some of these functions."

[35] I part company with Hitchens when he energetically mocks believers. One thing he doesn't account for in the life of the believer is the word "because." Believers do not worship or call on God for no reason and to no effect; we do so because of because. The Psalmist sang:

> I love the Lord *because* He hath heard my voice and my supplications.
> *Because* He hath inclined his ear unto me, therefore will I call upon Him as long
> as I live" (116:1, 2)

[36] Hitchens, Christopher. *Letters to a Young Contrarian*, Basic Books, a member of the Perseus Books Group, 2001